IMMUNOSUPPRESSION UNDER TRIAL

Transplantation and Clinical Immunology

Symposia Fondation Marcel Mérieux

VOLUME 31

Immunosuppression under Trial

Proceedings of the 31st Conference on
Transplantation and Clinical Immunology,
3 – 4 June, 1999

Edited by

P. Cochat

J. Traeger

C. Merieux

M. Derchavane

SPRINGER-SCIENCE+BUSINESS MEDIA, B.V.

A C.I.P. Catalogue record for this book is available from the Library of Congress

ISBN 978-94-010-5960-2   ISBN 978-94-011-4643-2 (eBook)
DOI 10.1007/978-94-011-4643-2

Printed on acid-free paper

Table of contents

List of contributors

D. ABRAMOWICZ
Nephrology Department
Hôpital Erasme
808 route de Lennik
B-1070 Bruxelles
Belgium

J. ALSINA
Servei de Nefrologia
Hospital de Bellvitge
Feixa llarga s/n
Hospitalet del Llobregat
E-08907 Barcelona
Spain

M. ANTOINE
Hôpital Erasme
Université Libre de Bruxelles
Département de Chirurgie
  Cardiaque
808 route de Lennik
B-1070 Bruxelles
Belgium

S. DE GEEST
Center for Health Services and
  Nursing Research
School of Public Health
Catholic University of Leuven
Kapucijnenvoer 35
B-3000 Leuven
Belgium

J.-M. DUBERNARD
Service d'Urologie et de Chirurgie de
  la Transplantation
Hôpital Edouard Herriot
F-69437 Lyon Cedex 03
France

O. FARGES
Service de Chirurgie Digestive et de
  Transplantation Hépatique
Hôpital Beaujon
100 Boulevard du Général Leclerc
F-92118 Clichy
France

J. HUTTON
MEDTAP International
27 Gilbert Street
London
W1Y 1RL
UK

B.L. KASISKE
Department of Medicine
Hennepin County Medical Center
701 Park Avenue South
Minneapolis
MN 55415
USA

P. LANDAIS
Service de Biostatistique et
  d'Informatique Médicale
Hôpital Necker Enfants Malades
149 rue de Sèvres
F-75743 Paris Cedex 15
France

C. LEGENDRE
Hôpital Saint-Louis
Service de Néphrologie
1 avenue Claude Vellefaux
F-75010 Paris
France

X. MARTIN
Service d'Urologie et Chirurgie de la
  Transplantation
Hôpital Edouard Herriot
F-69437 Lyon Cedex 03
France

Z.A. MASSY
INSERM U 507
Hôpital Necker
161 Rue de Sevres
F-75743 Paris Cedex 15
France

G. OPELZ
Institute of Immunology
University of Heidelberg
Im Neuenheimer Feld 305
D-69120 Heidelberg
Germany

J.-P. REVILLARD
Hôpital Edouard Herriot
Pavillon P
5 Place d'Arsonval
F-69437 Lyon
France

E. RITZ
Department of Internal Medicine
University of Heidelberg
Bergheimer Strasse 58
D-69115 Heidelberg
Germany

J.-S. SOULILLOU
ITERT-INSERM U437
CHU-Hotel Dieu
30 Bd. Jean Monnet
F-44093 Nantes
France

B. TÖNSHOFF
Division of Pediatric Nephrology
University Children's Hospital
Im Neuenheimer Feld 150
D-69120 Heidelberg
Germany

C. VAN BUREN
University of Texas School of
  Medicine
6431 Fannin, MSB 6.240
Houston
TX 77030
USA

Organizing Committee, Lyon

P. Cochat
President CITIC 1999

J. Traeger
J.L. Touraine
J.M. Dubernard
H. Betuel
J.P. Revillard
O. Bastien
R. Boulieu
J.J. Colpart
A. Lachaux
N. Lefrancois
X. Martin
J.F. Mornex
J.F. Obadia
C. Pouteil-Noble
V. Lachat
C. Dupuy

International Advisory Committee

J. Alsina, *Barcelona*
D. Forti, *Milano*
M. Goldman, *Bruxelles*
P. Lang, *Paris*
P. Morris, *Oxford*
G. Opelz, *Heidelberg*
G. Segoloni, *Torino*

PART ONE

Setting the stages in clinical trials

1. Current results as reference for future improvements in immunosuppression

G. OPELZ, B. DÖHLER AND T. WUJCIAK for the Collaborative
Transplant Study

Introduction

The immunosuppressive drug regimen most commonly used for kidney transplant recipients during the last 10 years was a combination of cyclosporine with either steroids or azathioprine, or both. More recently, new immunosuppressive drugs, such as tacrolimus, mycophenolate and rapamycin have been introduced and hopes were raised that these new medications would improve the success rate of kidney grafts. Experience with these new drugs is still limited and long-term follow up is currently not available. The present report provides an overview of results obtained with regimens that were considered 'standard' during the last 10 years. They should serve as a reference against which future improvements can be measured.

Methods

First cadaver kidney transplants performed from 1985 to 1995 and reported to the Collaborative Transplant Study by 305 centers in 46 countries were analyzed. The initial immunosuppressive regimen was recorded and analyzed according to the 'intention to treat' principle, except for the analysis in which 1-year maintenance regimens are specified. Graft outcome was recorded at 3, 6 and 12 months, and yearly thereafter. Graft survival rates were computed according to the Kaplan–Meier method. No exclusions were made and patients who died were counted as graft failures.

Results

Figure 1 shows graft survival rates for subgroups of patients who received various combinations of immunosuppressive drugs. A clear benefit of all cyclosporine regimens over the steroid and azathioprine regimen is evident (log rank $p < 0.0001$). Among the cyclosporine regimens, steroid-free combinations resulted in a slightly better result than regimens containing steroids. The same data plotted on semi-logarithmic scale show that the half-life estimates for long-term risk after the first post-transplant year are very similar for all regimens (Figure 2).

P. Cochat et al. (eds.), Immunosuppression under Trial, 3–9
©*1999 Kluwer Academic Publishers.*

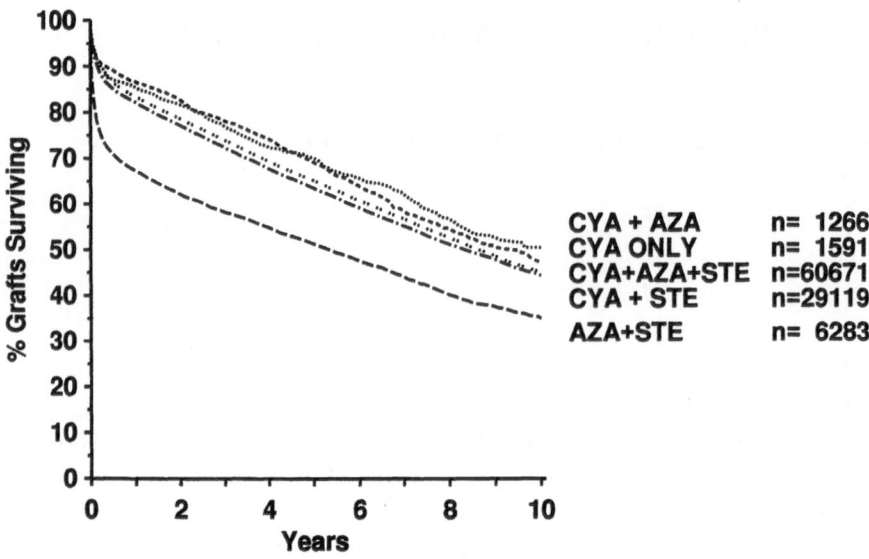

Fig. 1. Survival of first cadaver kidney transplants according to the initial (intention to treat) immunosuppressive drug regimen. Combinations of drugs and numbers of patients studied are indicated at end of each curve. CYA, cyclosporine; AZA, azathioprine; STE, steroids.

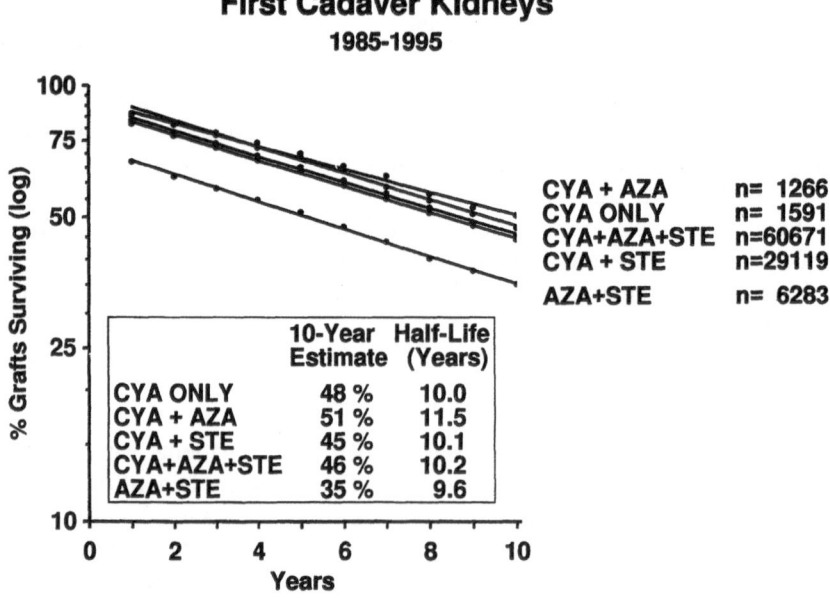

Fig. 2. Same results as shown in Figure 1, here plotted on semi-logarithmic scale to indicate risk rates of chronic graft loss. Estimated 10-year graft survival rates and half-lives are shown in box.

Although it has often been stated that no improvement in the long-term half-life of kidney transplants has been achieved during the last 15 years, the Collaborative Transplant Study data in fact show a substantial improvement when the first 3 study years are compared with the last 3 study years of the present analysis. Transplants performed between 1993 and 1995 had a strikingly better half-life time of 14.6 years, compared with a 9.3 year half-life time for transplants performed between 1985 and 1987 (Figure 3). Remarkably, these results were achieved in patients who were all on cyclosporine regimens, suggesting that perhaps a more diligent use of immunosuppressive drugs, in combination with other improvements related to better clinical care, may have contributed to the better success rate in recent years. One should also bear in mind that the improvement was achieved in spite of a tendency to expand the acceptance criteria for patients and donors who would not have been transplanted 10 or 15 years earlier because they would have been considered poor risks.

A clue concerning the important influence of maintenance immuno-suppression on long-term graft outcome is provided by the results shown in Figure 4. In patients who were on a cyclosporine + steroid + azathioprine triple-therapy regimen initially, the long-term curves separated when different maintenance regimens were compared. The best half-life performance was obtained with the two steroid-free cyclosporine maintenance regimens. The steroid-containing regimens resulted in shorter half-lives (Figure 4). Because it could be argued that patients on steroid-free maintenance might be those who did particularly well during the first post-transplant year, whereas patients on maintenance steroids might have had rejection problems and impaired graft function, a separate analysis was performed in patients who had excellent graft function at 1 year, as indicated by a serum creatinine value of <130 μmol/l. This analysis confirms the superior long-term outcome of patients on steroid-free maintenance immunosuppressive therapy with cyclosporine (Figure 5).

An important negative side effect of immunosuppressive treatment is the increased incidence of malignant tumors in transplant recipients. The incidence of tumors for the three most common immunosuppressive regimens (intention to treat) are depicted in Figure 6. Compared with the expected tumor rates in the background population, all three regimens produced an increase of malignant tumors (skin cancers were excluded) by approximately a factor of 2 (Figure 6).

Discussion

The introduction of cyclosporine for immunosuppression has resulted in a striking decline of the early post-transplant rejection rate (Figure 1). With cyclosporine-based immunosuppression, one can currently expect a 1-year function rate of approximately 85% for primary cadaver kidney transplants.

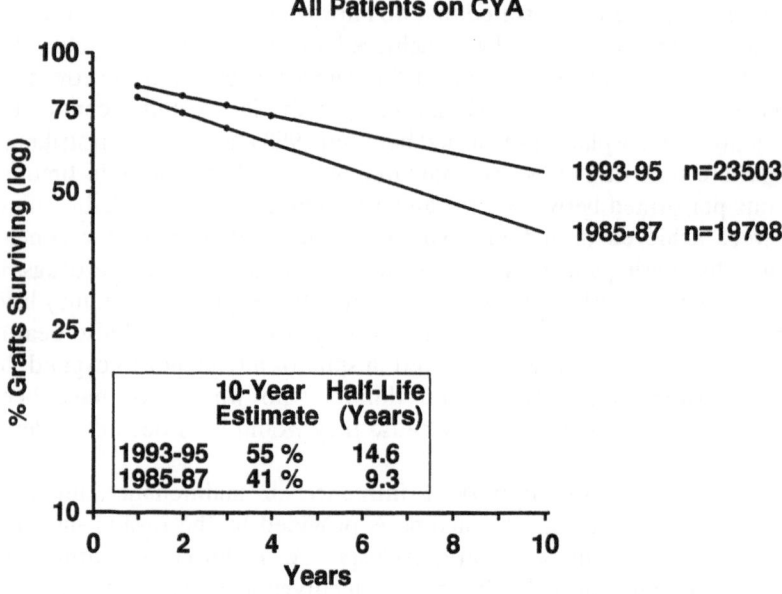

Fig. 3. Long-term risk comparison between transplants performed between 1985 and 1987 and 1993 and 1995. All patients were on cyclosporine-based immunosuppression. More recently performed transplants had a markedly improved long-term half-life.

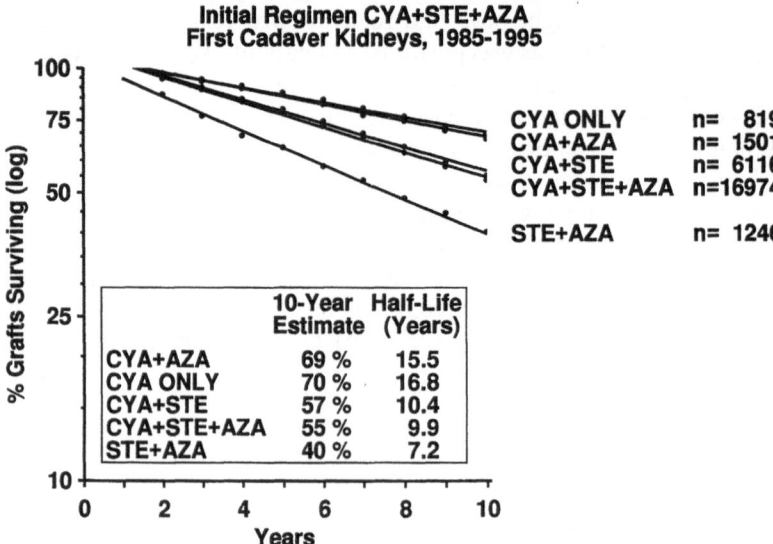

Fig. 4. Influence on maintenance immunosuppressive regimen administered at 1 year. All patients were initially on triple drug therapy, including cyclosporine, steroids, and azathioprine (CYA+STE+AZA). Ten-year survival estimates and half-life times are shown in box. Steroid-free maintenance therapy on cyclosporine resulted in the best long-term outcome.

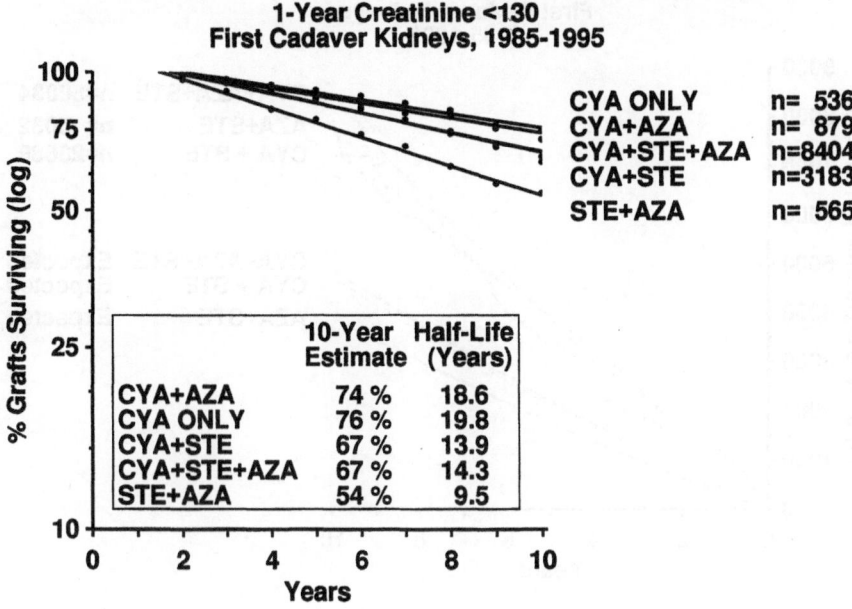

1-YEAR MAINTENANCE IMMUNOSUPPRESSION
1-Year Creatinine <130
First Cadaver Kidneys, 1985-1995

CYA ONLY	n=	536
CYA+AZA	n=	879
CYA+STE+AZA	n=	8404
CYA+STE	n=	3183
STE+AZA	n=	565

	10-Year Estimate	Half-Life (Years)
CYA+AZA	74 %	18.6
CYA ONLY	76 %	19.8
CYA+STE	67 %	13.9
CYA+STE+AZA	67 %	14.3
STE+AZA	54 %	9.5

Fig. 5. Same analysis as shown in Figure 4, here for a subset of patients who had excellent graft function at 1 year as indicated by a serum creatinine value of <130 μmol/l.

Naturally, attempts must be made to reduce the early rate of graft loss even further. Literature reports indicate that the incidence of acute rejection episodes after transplantation can be reduced with the use of new pharmacological drugs as well as with polyclonal or monoclonal antibody induction treatment. Whether a lower rate of rejection translates into improved long-term outcome, however, is presently unclear.

The main challenge for the next decade will be to improve the half-life for the period following the first post-transplant year. Figure 2 shows that the improvement in graft survival attributable to the introduction of cyclosporine has not resulted in a markedly better half-life slope compared with the traditional azathioprine and steroid regimen. The 1993–1995 data shown in Figure 3, on the other hand, suggest that, even without the use of new drugs, the probability for good long-term outcome has improved in recently transplanted patients. New immunosuppressive drugs, or regimens containing combinations of new drugs will, therefore, have to be measured against this current background of a long-term half-life of nearly 15 years.

Steroid-free maintenance immunosuppression is a promising option that probably can be taken advantage of in a large fraction of patients. A prospec-

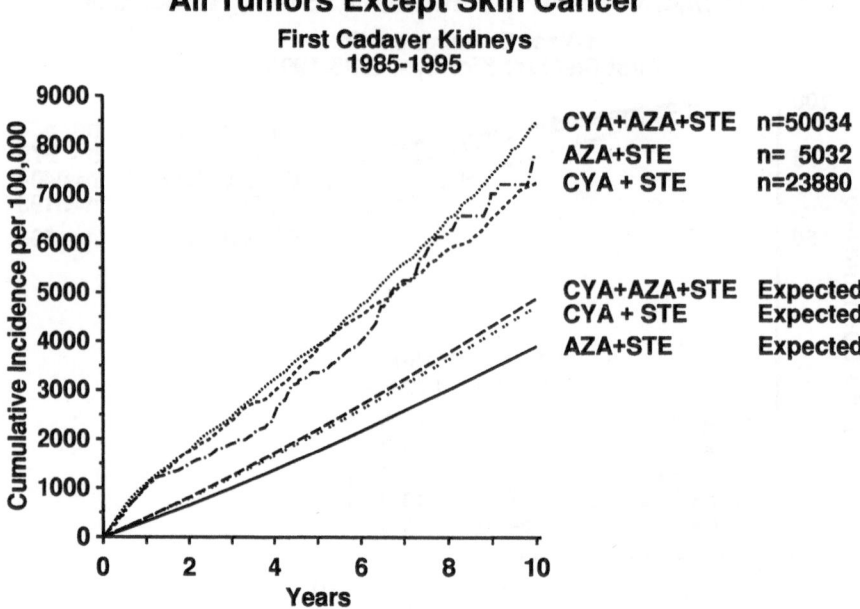

Fig. 6.   Incidence of malignant tumors in recipients of first cadaver kidney transplants. Skin cancers were excluded from this analysis. The combinations of immunosuppressive drugs administered (intention to treat) as well as the numbers of patients studied are indicated at end of each curve. The 'expected' reference rate was computed using reference registry data (Cancer Incidence in five Continents), standardized for each subgroup according to recipient age, gender and geographical origin.

tive study of steroid withdrawal which is currently underway within the framework of the Collaborative Transplant Study shows that, in more than 500 patients, the rate of successful steroid weaning was 75%, and that after 3 years of follow up there was no perceptible deleterious effect of steroid withdrawal (Collaborative Transplant Study Newsletter, February 1999).

The data on the increased incidence of malignant tumors in transplant recipients should serve as a warning sign. More potent immunosuppression might further promote the occurrence of malignancies. Tumors such as non-Hodgin lymphoma and Kaposi sarcoma are seen at strikingly increased frequencies even early after transplantation, whereas other tumors may occur only after years of exposure to immunosuppressive drugs. An important goal of the Collaborative Transplant Study is the establishment of valid incidence rates for various tumors in a large population of transplant recipients. The tumor rates observed with new immunosuppressive drugs will have to be monitored carefully and compared with established standards in order to detect any deleterious trends as early as possible.

Acknowledgement

The generous support of 305 transplant centers participating in the Collaborative Transplant Study is gratefully acknowledged. This work was supported in part by a grant from Deutsche Krebshilfe, Bonn, Germany.

2. Rationale of clinical trials from the physician

C. LEGENDRE

Clinical trials have been used to assess the efficacy of therapeutic and preventive interventions in human subjects for more than two centuries. Clinical trial design, study implementation methods and analytical techniques have been refined progressively to make the clinical trial the 'gold standard' for both clinical and epidemiologic researchers. In transplantation, as well as in other fields, the criteria for a meaningful clinical trial are straightforward. We will briefly review these criteria as well as the current rationale of clinical trials in organ transplantation with a special reference to kidney transplantation.

First, of course, the investigator set a key question. The importance of this question depends mainly on its clinical and public health relevance. At the end of the 1970s, when cyclosporine A was first introduced, the main question to be asked in kidney transplantation was whether it was possible to improve graft survival rate, especially in the short-term. In the European Multicentre study reported in 1993 [1], the authors were able to demonstrate that under cyclosporine A immunosuppression, 1-year graft survival rate improved from 52 to 72%, a difference which was highly significant ($p < 0.001$). Since then it has not been possible to demonstrate such a tremendous short-term benefit with any new immunosuppressive drug, namely mycophenolate mofetil [2] or tacrolimus [3].

The important question therefore had to change in order to ascertain differences between immunosuppressants. If it is not possible to improve 1-year graft survival rate, it might be possible to decrease the incidence of early acute rejection, which was considered as a relevant surrogate marker. Indeed, several new immunosuppressive drugs did so: mycophenolate mofetil [2], tacrolimus [3], OKT3® [4], and anti-IL2 receptor monoclonal antibodies [5]. It is likely that it is no longer the case. In 1998, at the American Society of Transplant Physicians, some of the most recent studies were unable to show any difference in acute rejection rate between two immunosuppressive protocols [6].

It is still possible, however, to show that the incidence of severe acute rejection (grade III according to the Banff classification) is significantly decreased in patients receiving tacrolimus-based immunosuppression compared with those on cyclosporine-based immunosuppression. Decreasing the incidence and severity of acute rejection remains a significant and relevant issue in organ transplantation, but it has become very difficult and even unrealistic to set up a trial designed to demonstrate a statistically significant difference: the number

P. Cochat et al. (eds.), Immunosuppression under Trial, 11–13
©1999 Kluwer Academic Publishers.

of patients to be included is just too big. It is then very important that rapamycine and its derivative, SDZ-RAD are going to be introduced on the immunosuppressive market, as drugs which are not superior but equivalent to pre-existing drugs with regard to immunosuppressive potency.

What then, are the important questions which are to be asked at the end of the century in kidney transplantation? As transplant physicians and surgeons are now perfectly aware of long-term deleterious complications of immunosuppressive drugs, clinical trials must be designed to define how to decrease their incidence and severity. Long-term metabolic complications include post-transplant diabetes mellitus [7], dyslipidemia [8], osteopenia [9] and 'metabolic risk factor syndrome' [10]. As a consequence, immuno-suppressive drugs must now be compared with regard to their overall tolerance profile and clinical trials will have to be designed for such comparisons.

Another important long-term issue is the incidence of cancer which parallels the burden of immunosuppression. However, it is only recently that Dantal et al. [11] demonstrated in a very important study that it was possible to decrease significantly the incidence of cancer if the immunosuppressive 'load' was decreased.

The influence of immunosuppression on long-term results of transplantation, and particularly on the incidence of 'chronic rejection' or better, chronic allograft nephropathy, is also of utmost importance. Although during the past years significant improvement have been made toward understanding immuno-suppression and identifying immunological and non-immunological factors that increase the overall risk of developing chronic allograft nephropathy [12], no significant therapeutic improvement has been noted. As a history of acute rejection has been established as a major risk factor for subsequent renal allograft loss, it was logical to think that decreasing the incidence of acute rejection would lead to a decreased incidence rate of chronic rejection. However, the mycophenolate mofetil study [13] was rather disappointing, since 3-year graft survival rate was similar whatever the incidence of acute rejection. This study was unfortunately not designed to answer such a long-term issue which therefore remains to be evaluated.

Other issues have to be addressed. Is it possible to stop steroids and when is it still useful to use anti-lymphocyte antibodies? is it possible to interrupt cyclosporine and what molecule is going to replace it? are anti-LFA1 antibodies able to prevent delayed graft function? is cytomegalovirus infection preventable? etc.

For some time, it has been possible to give an adequate answer to a relevant question in kidney transplantation with the help of a new immunosuppressive drug. As the number of available immunosuppressive drugs is constantly growing, it is no longer possible to clarify complex issues with such an approach. In recent years, the transplant community has been enjoying unprecedented improvements in short-term renal allograft survival rates. Current relevant questions appear to be much more complex to address because of their multifactorial nature. It is therefore a very difficult challenge to develop and test strategies aimed at minimizing long-term risks of immunosuppression.

References

1. European Multicentre Trial Group. Cyclosporin in cadaveric renal transplantation: one-year follow-up of a multicentre trial. Lancet. 1983; 2: 986–989.
2. European Mycophenolate Mofetil Cooperative Study Group. Placebo-controlled study of mycophenolate mofetil combined with cyclosporin and corticosteroids for prevention of acute rejection. Lancet. 1995; 345: 1321–1325.
3. Mayer AD, Dmitrewski J, Squifflet JP et al. Multicenter randomized trial comparing tacrolimus (FK506) and cyclosporine in the prevention of renal allograft rejection. Transplantation. 1997; 64: 436–443.
4. Norman DJ, Kahana L, Stuart FP et al. A randomized clinical trial of induction therapy with OKT3 in kidney transplantation. Transplantation. 1993; 55: 44–50.
5. Nashan B, Moore R, Amlot P et al. Randomised trial of basiliximab versus placebo for control of acute cellular rejection in renal allograft recipients. Lancet. 1997; 351: 1193–1198.
6. Yang HC, Holman MJ, Ulsh PJ et al. Tacrolimus 'low dose'/mycophenolate mofetil versus micro-emulsion cyclosporine/'low dose' mycophenolate mofetil after kidney transplantation. One-year follow-up of a prospective randomized clinical trial. Am. Soc. Transpl. Phys., Chicago 1998, [abstract].
7. Krentz AJ, Dmitrewski J, Mayer D et al. Effects of immunosuppressive agents on glucose metabolism. Clin. Immunother. 1995; 4: 103–123.
8. Massy ZA, Kasiske BL. Post-transplant hyperlipidemia: mechanisms and management. J. Am. Soc. Nephrol. 1996; 7: 971–977
9. Massari PU. Disorders of bone and mineral metabolism after renal transplantation. Kidney Int. 1997; 52: 1412–1421.
10. Dimeny E, Fellström B. Metabolic abnormalities in renal transplant recipients. Risk factors and predictors of chronic graft dysfunction. Nephrol. Dial. Transplant. 1997; 12: 21–24.
11. Dantal J, Hourmant M, Cantarovich D et al. Effect of long-term immunosuppression in kidney-graft recipients on cancer incidence: randomised comparison of two cyclosporin regimens. Lancet. 1998; 351: 623–628.
12. Monaco AP, Burke JF, Ferguson RM et al. Current thinking on chronic renal allograft rejection: issues, concerns, and recommendations from a 1977 roundtable discussion. Am. J. Kidney Dis. 1999; 33: 150–160.
13. Mathew TH, for the Tricontinental Mycophenolate Mofetil Renal Transplantation Study Group. A blinded, long-term, randomized multicenter study of mycophenalate mofetil in cadaveric renal transplantation: results at 3 years. Transplantation. 1998; 65: 1450–1454.

3. Minimal standards for reporting clinical trial results in transplantation

B. L. KASISKE and H. CHAKKERA

Introduction

A clinical trial is a planned (prospective) experiment in which individuals receive the same or similar therapy in order to determine the risk and/or benefit of that therapy. Not all therapeutic decisions in medicine are based on the results of clinical trials. For example, insulin is the standard treatment of diabetic ketoacidosis, even though this therapy was never tested in a randomized controlled trial. Similarly, the need to use immunosuppression in organ transplantation (excepting transplants between identical twins) was not established by clinical trials. However, virtually every other decision regarding immunosuppression has subsequently been subjected to rigorous testing in clinical trials. Thus, the importance of clinical trials in transplantation is self-evident.

The strength of evidence supporting the use of a therapy is based on both the quality of clinical trials testing the therapy, and the quality of the reporting of the trial results. A clinical trial that is not reported is useless, or even worse than useless if it contributes to publication bias. Similarly, a clinical trial that fails to adequately report its methods can be counterproductive if clinicians thereby misjudge the strength of the results. From a practical standpoint, the quality of a study can be no better than the quality of its reporting. In a quality assessment of breast cancer treatment trials, Liberati and co-workers made a distinction between 'internal validity' and 'external validity' [1]. Internal validity referred to the quality of the study design and execution, while external validity referred to the reporting of information required to determine its generalizability. They contacted authors when information was incomplete or ambiguous and found that the external validity scores increased after doing so. They concluded that the studies were better than the reports indicated. However, because it is not always possible for readers to contact authors, and because the information provided informally by authors may not be 100% accurate (for several reasons), a strong argument can be made that reports of clinical trials should be considered only as good as the information provided in the published, peer-reviewed account.

What constitutes quality in clinical trials and their reporting has been the subject of many reviews and editorials. Formal and informal, semiquantitative

P. Cochat et al. (eds.), Immunosuppression under Trial, 15–24
©1999 Kluwer Academic Publishers.

and qualitative methods for assessing the quality of clinical trials have been developed [2–6]. Although it may seem intuitively obvious, whether quality matters has only recently been studied systematically. Emerson and co-workers empirically examined the role of study quality in seven meta-analyses and found no relation between quality scores and treatment effects [7]. On the other hand, Kahn and colleagues conducted a meta-analysis of 149 trials examining anti-estrogen therapy in men with oligospermia and blindly assessed that quality of each trial [8]. They found that poor quality studies produced positive results, whereas high-quality studies found no benefit. They concluded that methodologically poor studies tended to exaggerate the treatment effect. More recently, Moher and co-workers examined the effect of quality in 11 randomly selected meta-analyses [9]. They found that low quality trials were associated with an increased estimate of benefit. Similarly, Schultz and co-workers found that inadequate concealment was associated with reports of larger effects of treatment [10]. Thus, most evidence suggests that quality can affect the reported results of randomized controlled trials.

Features of quality in reports of clinical trials

Ethics statement

How patient rights were protected should be clearly described. Reports should indicate any approvals that were obtained by institutional review boards. It should also be stated that in every case informed consent was obtained.

Sponsorship disclosure

Investigations supported by companies that may profit from the use of the therapies studied may be subject to publication bias and other biases. Rochon and co-workers examined the effect of study sponsorship on study results reported in trials of non-steroidal anti-inflammatory drugs [11]. Reviewers who were blinded to manufacturer status evaluated the narrative interpretation of results and extracted data from 81 randomized controlled trials. Among the 72 manufacturer-sponsored studies, the investigators found that the manufacturer-associated drug was almost always reported to be equal or superior in efficacy and toxicity than the comparison drug. They concluded that there may be selective publication and/or biased interpretation of results of manufacturer-associated trials. Thus, it is important that reports of clinical trials clearly indicate the sponsor of the study.

Describing the study population

The number of study participants who were included in other reports should be clearly indicated. It is surprising how often data that have previously been reported in one way or another are reported again, without mention of the prior publication. Data are sometimes published a second or third time with additional patients, additional follow-up, both additional patients and follow-up, or neither. This seems to be particularly true of literature in transplantation, where publications are often required for participation in scientific meetings, and appear after only cursory peer review in *Transplantation Proceedings*. Many, but not all of these studies are then reported again in peer-reviewed journals. Any duplication or overlap should be clearly indicated. Otherwise, the readers' only option is to compare descriptions of study designs and patient populations, and thereby surmise from close similarities that there is duplication.

The report should clearly indicate how patients were selected. Specific inclusion and exclusion criteria should be described, and the number of patients in the population who met the inclusion and exclusion criteria should be indicated. In addition, the number of patients who refused to participate, and the number of patients who withdrew after randomization should be indicated. The chances for bias increase if the proportion of patients who choose not to participate is high. In addition, the generalizability of the results may be questioned if only a minority of patients participates.

Whether the number of patients included in the trial was predetermined should be indicated. In addition, how the number of study patients was determined should be described. No doubt some trials enroll patients until the investigators fatigue or the financial support for the study runs out. However, if the number of subjects was based on statistical calculations, then the report should indicate what assumptions were made regarding alpha (*p*-value), power ($=1-\beta$), and the expected magnitude of the treatment differences.

The population from which patients were recruited, and how they were recruited, should also be described. Studies that do not systematically recruit all of the patients in a defined population may be subject to selection bias. It is common for nurses and clinicians to look for patients who they believe 'will be good for the study' and vice versa. Such recruitment biases are probably less likely if all patients within a defined population are asked to participate. All pertinent patient characteristics should be separately reported by treatment and control groups, with appropriate statistics to test differences between the groups. Basic demographic features, such as age, gender, and race should be included, as well as any patient characteristics that could influence the results, e.g. donor source and incidence of delayed graft function.

Describing therapies

Any aspects of therapy that could influence the results should be described. In the case of immunosuppression, the dose and dosing interval should be indicated. Equally detailed information should be given concerning any other immunosuppression that was used during the period of study.

Basic study design

It is well established that the design of a study has a major influence on the strength of evidence that its results provide. It is critical, therefore, to clearly describe the study design. This description should indicate whether the trial was a prospective, clinical trial or a retrospective, observational study. All too often the description of the trial is ambiguous and readers are left to speculate on the true nature of the study design. A common error is for authors to simply state that a measurement was made before and after treatment, without indicating whether the data were obtained in a retrospective chart review or in a prospective clinical trial. In general, it is probably best to assume that the data were obtained in a retrospective fashion if it is not clearly stated that a prospective, clinical trial was conducted.

How the study was controlled is a critical piece of information for assessing quality, and this should be clearly described. One of the major pitfalls of clinical trials is the tendency for high values to decline and low values to increase, even without treatment. This 'tendency-to-the-mean' effect can only be adequately controlled in a parallel-group, randomized, controlled trial. In some studies, patients serve as their own controls, and measurements are made before and after treatment. Most would consider such a study to be uncontrolled, and very susceptible to tendency-to-the-mean effects and other biases. In a cross-over study design, patients may be alternately observed with and without treatment. With cross-over studies authors should indicate what, if any, study design and/or analytical steps were taken to deal with possible residual, lingering effects of treatment that could cause the sequence of treatment to influence the results. In a parallel-group, study design, patients are assigned to one or more treatment and control groups, and then measurements are obtained prospectively from patients in each group. One type of parallel-group design, and the gold standard for all clinical trials, is the randomized, controlled trial.

Whether or not a wash-in period was used should be indicated. A wash-in period is particularly helpful in an otherwise uncontrolled trial, helping to negate tendency-to-the-mean effects that render the results of uncontrolled trials so unreliable. A wash-out period is also an important design feature of crossover studies, so that lingering effects of treatment can be reduced.

Finally, the length of follow-up that was planned should be indicated, as well as whether it was planned for all patients to be followed for the same length of time. Some trials follow all patients for the same length of time. Others may enroll patients in an on-going fashion, and follow patients for different lengths of time. In the latter case, it is important to describe this approach in the methods and to include an exact accounting of the duration of follow-up for all patients in the reporting of the results (discussed below).

Allocation to treatment and control groups

A critical defense against bias is random allocation into treatment and control groups. It is critical that the report describes exactly how patients were allocated to the study groups. Elements in that description should include how the random sequence was determined. Simply assigning every other patient to treatment or control is a common practice, but is not the same as random allocation. Any violations of the intended allocation process should also be described. It should be stated whether some patients were included even if they entered the study outside of the random allocation process. Occasionally patents may be enrolled in a randomized trial 'only if they can be randomized to the treatment group.' The frequency of such violations should be clearly indicated. Whether patients, investigators, or both were masked, or 'blinded' should be indicated. Specific reasons why masking was not possible should be stated. Finally, any attempts to assess compliance with therapy should be indicated.

Data analysis

How the data were analyzed should be clearly described. The statistical tests for differences that were used should be indicated along with a brief statement of the rationale for their selection. Which tests were used for which end-points should be made clear. What was done to handle withdrawals should be described. Did the analysis include all patients who entered the trial (by intention to treat), were only those patients who stayed on the treatment regimen included, or were data analyzed with both methods? How were cross-overs handled? When more than one end-point was used, what steps were taken to account for multiple 'looks' at the data.

Presenting results

It is critically important to report the results in a clear fashion. Investigators and editors should consider reporting results in such a way that their description allows easy, reproducible extraction for comparing and combining with the results of other, similar studies in a meta-analysis. Ideally, individual data should be reported. This should be strongly encouraged when the number of patients is not prohibitively large, e.g. less than 50. When reporting individual patient data is not practical, then summary results should be reported in as much detail as possible.

End-points in clinical trials of renal transplant recipients are often appropriately described as the time to an event, or the survival free of an event, such as death or graft failure. When this is the case, adequate reporting is crucial. It is not enough to simply report the proportion of patients who survived during a mean, or median, duration of follow-up. Kaplan–Meier survival curves are usually adequate if enough information is included. Along with the survival curves, the number of patients entering each time interval of follow-up should be indicated. It is helpful to also display the actual proportions surviving at discrete intervals (Figure 1). It may also be appropriate to report results as both absolute and relative risk reduction, as well as the number needed to treat to spare one event. If there are unavoidable differences between the study groups, then results should be reported with and without statistical adjustment for these differences. Finally, a comprehensive accounting of the type and frequency of adverse events should be reported.

Key elements in the discussion

The discussion should be brief and to the point. The medical literature would be well served if more data and less speculation were reported. Ideally, each randomized, controlled trial should be reported along with a cumulative meta-analysis that included data from similar, previously reported trials. In this way the study results could be quantitatively compared to the results of previous studies. Although this is not practical, the authors should at least compare their results with those of all previous, similar trials in a qualitative fashion. This can

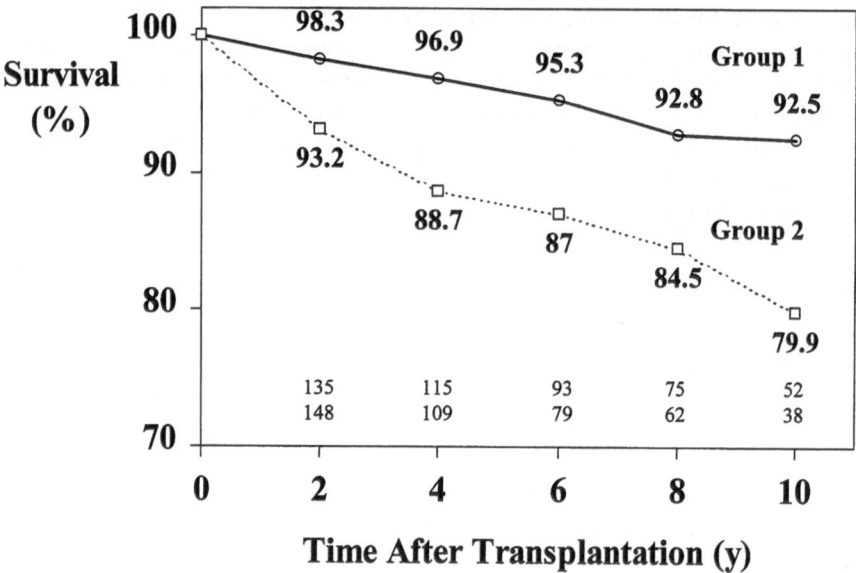

Fig, 1.   Example of a Kaplan–Meier plot of survival data. The legend could be a brief description of group 1 and group 2 and the number of patients in each group at time 0. The p-value could be included in the legend (or in the figure itself), along with how the p-value was derived, e.g., by the log-rank test. The legend should also indicate that the number of patients surviving at each time interval is indicated by the numbers above the x-axis for group 1 (upper row) and group 2 (lower row).

be done succinctly. If there are many such trials, a table can be used to summarize their results. Reasons for similarities and differences in the results of the trials can be addressed (Table 1).

Quality of controlled trials of cyclosporine withdrawal in renal transplantation

To provide an illustrative example of the quality of studies and their reporting in renal transplantation, we reviewed clinical trials that investigated cyclosporine withdrawal strategies in renal transplant recipients. We searched Medline and bibliographies of published trials and reviews. We included only controlled, clinical trials. We excluded retrospective, observational studies. We arbitrarily selected a number of easily codifiable parameters that reflect both study quality and its reporting.

We located 15 controlled trials [12–26]. Eight of these reports were published in regular, peer-reviewed journals, while 7 were published in *Transplantation Proceedings* (Table 2). Several quality indicators appeared to be more prevalent among studies published in peer-reviewed journals (Table 2). Only three of the 15 reports indicated that the study had been approved by an institutional review board and only three indicated the source of funding. Only two studies indicated that a sample size estimate had been used to select the number of patients enrolled in the study. Nine studies reported inclusion and exclusion criteria, and 10 indicated important patient characteristics by study groups. All 15 studies used a parallel-group design, and 14 allocated patients randomly. However, only four clearly described the randomization process. This failure to clearly describe the randomization process is problematic. In two instances, for example, patients were said to be 'consecutively randomized' leaving it unclear whether true random allocation was carried out, or a pseudo-random allocation (where every other patient was assigned to withdrawal versus control groups) was employed. In eight reports the statistical tests used to assess differences in outcomes were not clearly described, and in three studies the results for major end-points, e.g., graft survival, were not clearly reported. Altogether, this exercise demonstrated that there is much room for improvement in the reporting of clinical trial results in renal transplantation. These results are similar to those previously reported in the general medical literature [27].

Summary

There is a growing awareness that the quality of a study and its presentation influence its reported outcome. As in other areas of medicine, reports of clinical trials in renal transplantation are often of poor quality. Guidelines and checklists are available that can help investigators improve the quality of clinical trial reporting. Both authors and journal editors should make a greater effort in improving the quality of reporting of clinical trial results. Better

Table 1.   Check-list of clinical trial features

Ethics
Institutional review
Informed consent

Sponsorship
Support from private corporations
Support from public sources

Study Population
Overlap or duplication
Inclusion and exclusion criteria
Number meeting inclusion/exclusion criteria
Number refusing and withdrawing
How the sample size was determined
Who was or was not recruited
Patient characteristics (by treatment group)

Therapies
Dose and dosing intervals, etc.
Important ancillary therapies in all groups

Study Design Features
Prospective or retrospective
Simple before/after treatment (uncontrolled)
Crossover design
Parallel groups
Wash-in period
Wash-out (especially in crossover designs)
Length of follow-up

Allocation of Patients
Randomization methods
Blinded patients/investigators

Data Analysis
Statistical tests
Intent-to-treat analysis
Handling multiple looks

Results
Number of patients in each follow-up time interval
Exact survival in each follow-up time interval
Absolute and relative risk reduction
Number needed to treat
Adverse events

Discussion
Adequate review of other pertinent trials

Table 2. Quality features in reports of controlled trials studying cyclosporine withdrawal after renal transplantation

Clinical trial features	Number of Trials		
	Total ($n = 15$)	Peer Reviewed No (7)	Yes (8)
Published in a peer-reviewed journal	8	–	–
Institutional review/informed consent described	3	0	3
Source of support clearly acknowledged	3	0	3
Statistical calculations determined sample size	2	1	1
Inclusion/exclusion criteria clearly indicated	9	3	6
Important patient characteristics reported by group	10	4	6
Parallel treatment/control group design used	15	7	8
Random allocation to study groups used	14	6	8
Randomization process clearly described	4	1	3
Statistical tests clearly described	7	0	7
Endpoints reported precisely	12	6	6

reporting of results may directly and indirectly lead to a more efficient use of clinical trials in renal transplantation.

References

1. Liberati A, Himel HN, Chalmers TC. A quality assessment of randomized control trials of primary treatment of breast cancer. J. Clin. Oncol. 1986; 4: 942–951.
2. Chalmers TC, Smith HJ, Blackburn B et al. A method for assessing the quality of a randomized control trial. Controlled Clin. Trials. 1981; 2: 31–49.
3. Oxman AD, Sackett DL, Guyatt GH. Users' guides to the medical literature. I. How to get started. The Evidence-Based Medicine Working Group. JAMA. 1993; 270: 2093–2095.
4. Moher D, Jadad AR, Tugwell P. Assessing the quality of randomized controlled trials. Current issues and future directions. Int. J. Technol. Assess. Health Care. 1996; 12: 195–208.
5. Jadad AR, Moore RA, Carroll D et al. Assessing the quality of reports of randomized clinical trials: is blinding necessary? Controlled Clin. Trials. 1996; 17: 1–12.
6. Begg C, Cho M, Eastwood S et al. Improving the quality of reporting of randomized controlled trials. The CONSORT statement. JAMA. 1996; 276: 637–639.
7. Emerson JD, Burdick E, Hoaglin DC, Mosteller F, Chalmers TC. An empirical study of the possible relation of treatment differences to quality scores in controlled randomized clinical trials. Controlled Clin. Trials. 1990; 11: 339–352.
8. Khan KS, Daya S, Jadad A. The importance of quality of primary studies in producing unbiased systematic reviews. Arch. Intern. Med. 1996; 156: 661–666.
9. Moher D, Pham B, Jones A et al. Does quality of reports of randomised trials affect estimates of intervention efficacy reported in meta-analyses? Lancet. 1998; 352: 609–613.
10. Schulz KF, Chalmers I, Hayes RJ, Altman DG. Empirical evidence of bias. Dimensions of methodological quality associated with estimates of treatment effects in controlled trials. JAMA. 1995; 273: 408–412.
11. Rochon PA, Gurwitz JH, Simms RW et al. A study of manufacturer-supported trials of nonsteroidal anti- inflammatory drugs in the treatment of arthritis. Arch. Intern. Med. 1994; 154: 157–163.
12. Land W, Castro LA, Hillebrand G, Günther K, Gokel JM. Conversion rejection consequences by changing the immunosuppressive therapy from cyclosporine to azathioprine after kidney

transplantation. Transplant. Proc. 1983; 15: 2857–2861.

13. Hoitsma AJ, Wetzels JFM, van Lier HJJ, Berden JHM, Koene RAP. Cyclosporin treatment with conversion after three months versus conventional immunosuppression in renal allograft recipients. Lancet. 1987; 1: 584–586.

14. Morris PJ, Chapman JR, Allen RD et al. Cyclosporin conversion versus conventional immunosuppression: long-term follow-up and histological evaluation. Lancet. 1987; 1: 586–591.

15. Spielberger M, Aigner F, Schmid T, Bösmüller C, Königsrainer A, Margreiter R. Long-term results of cadaveric renal transplantation after conversion from cyclosporine to azathioprine: a controlled randomized trial. Transplant. Proc. 1988; 20: 169–170.

16. Hall BM, Tiller DJ, Hardie I et al. Comparison of three immunosuppressive regimens in cadaver renal transplantation: long-term cyclosporine, short-term cyclosporine followed by azathioprine and prednisolone, and azathioprine and prednisolone without cyclosporine. N. Engl. J. Med. 1988; 318: 1499–1507.

17. Sagalowsky AI, Reisman ME, Dawidson I, Toto R, Peters PC, Helderman JH. Late cyclosporine conversion carried risk of irreversible rejection. Transplant. Proc. 1988; 20: 157–160.

18. Büsing M, Hölzer H, Schareck WD et al. Is long-term therapy without cyclosporin A (CsA) indispensable or dangerous? One-year results of a prospective randomized trial. Transplant. Proc. 1989; 21: 1601–1603.

19. Sweny P, Lui SF, Scoble JE, Varghese Z, Fernando ON, Moorhead JF. Conversion of stable renal allografts at one year from cyclosporin A to azathioprine: a randomized controlled study. Transplant. Int. 1990; 3: 19–22.

20. Hiesse C, Neyrat N, Deglise-Favre A et al. Randomized prospective trial of elective cyclosporine withdrawal from triple therapy at 6 months after cadaveric renal transplantation. Transplant. Proc. 1991; 23: 987–989.

21. Isoniemi HM, Ahonen J, Tikkanen MJ et al. Long-term consequences of different immuno-suppressive regimens for renal allografts. Transplantation. 1993; 55: 494–499.

22. Pedersen EB, Hansen HE, Kornerup HJ, Madsen S, Sørensen AWS. Long-term graft survival after conversion from cyclosporin to azathioprine 1 year after renal transplantation. A prospective, randomized study from 1 to 6 years after transplantation. Nephrol. Dial. Transplant. 1993; 8: 250–254.

23. Heering P, Westhoff A, Ivens K, Kutkuhn B, Grabensee B. Reduction of immunosuppressive therapy after renal transplantation: a randomized study. Transplant. Proc. 1994; 26: 2530–2532.

24. Delmonico FL, Tolkoff-Rubin M, Auchincloss H Jr et al. Management of the renal allograft recipient: Immunosuppressive protocols for long-term success. Clin. Transplant. 1994; 8: 34–39.

25. Hollander AAMJ, van Saase JLCM, Kootte AMM et al. Beneficial effects of conversion from cyclosporin to azathioprine after kidney transplantation. Lancet. 1995; 345: 610–614.

26. Saadi MG, Francis MR, Selim OE. Five-year follow-up of early post-renal transplantation cyclosporin withdrawal: Do we benefit from a state of tolerance? Transplant. Proc. 1997; 29: 2593–2595.

27. Moher D. CONSORT: An evolving tool to help improve the quality of reports of randomized controlled trials. JAMA. 1998; 279: 1489–1491.

4. Methodological approach of clinical trials for renal transplantation

P. LANDAIS AND J. P. JAIS

The search for more effective and less toxic immunosuppressive agents to control transplant rejection is a challenge. Clinical trials provide a framework to take on this challenge. As stated by Senn, there are five main purposes to a clinical trial summarized by a mnemonic using the five vowels: anticipation, ethics, inference, organization and utmost good faith [1]. Methodological issues in renal transplantation will be illustrated by recent publications.

Hypothesis testing

Choosing the hypotheses

The general procedure of hypothesis testing in clinical trials requires defining a null hypothesis (called H_0). The objective is to disprove this null hypothesis. The hypothesis might be, for example, that the efficacy of a new immunosuppressive agent is no different from the standard drug or from a placebo. It may be that the efficacy of a new strategy is not different from a standard strategy. The alternative hypothesis (called H_1) that we would like to demonstrate specifies that the new drug or the new strategy is different from the standard drug or strategy. Note that the alternative hypothesis corresponds to a multitude of situations where the difference between the experimental treatment and the standard treatment is different from zero. Practically, to plan a trial one must define a particular clinically relevant value, for the difference of effects between the two treatments, which will allow a power calculation. When choosing between H_0 and H_1, there is a risk involved. In fact it implies that either H_0 or H_1 is true. The choice between H_0 and H_1 is attached to a risk of failure quantified by two types of probability. The probability of rejecting H_0 when it is true is called α or a type I error. The probability of failing to reject the null hypothesis when it is in fact false is called β or a type II error. It is not possible to minimize simultaneously both types of errors. By convention, α is held at a given level, generally 0.05. It is therefore possible to look for the lowest level of β. The power of a test is defined as one minus β, given that H_1 is true. From these elements it appears that for a given value of α the power increases with a decreasing variation, an increasing difference between the treatments compared or with an increasing sample size (Figure 1).

P. Cochat et al. (eds.), Immunosuppression under Trial, 25–37
©1999 Kluwer Academic Publishers.

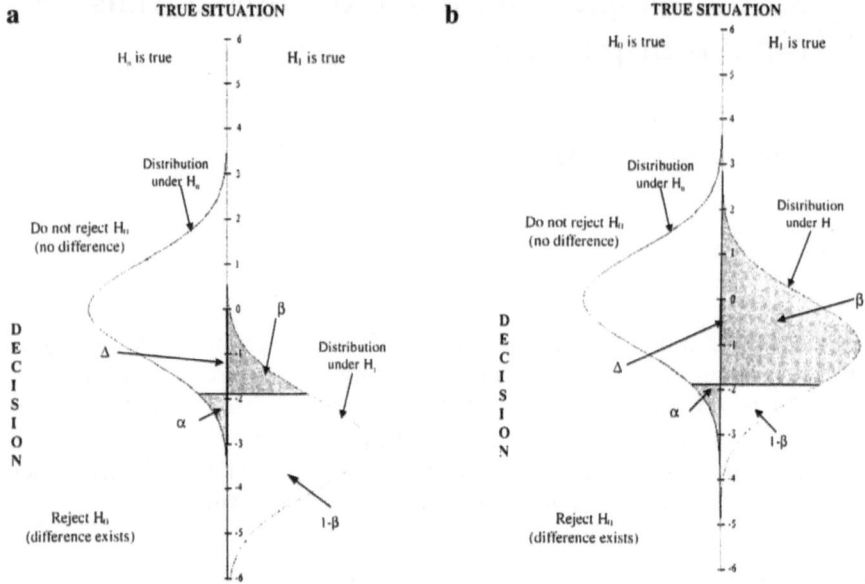

Fig. 1.   Modification of the expected difference between mean treatment effects (Δ) on the power of a test. (a) α, β and power (1 – β) considering the distribution under H_0 and under H_1 for a one-sided test, Δ is the difference means under H_0 and under H_1. (b) Given α is constant and the variance unchanged, when Δ decreases then (1 – β) decreases

P-value

The *P*-value is often wrongly interpreted as the probability that the null hypothesis is true. In fact, a *P*-value is the probability of observing a value as extreme or more extreme than the value observed, given that the null hypothesis is true. Given that the difference between two treatments may take an infinity of values, the probability to observe a difference exactly null between two treatments is infinitesimal.

The *P*-value is sometimes perceived as a measure of the weight of evidence of a statistical test: the lower the *P*-value, the greater the difference between two treatments. This is not appropriate. Let us observe the following two situations: a very low difference between two groups of thousands of patients on the one hand and an important difference between two groups of limited size on the other hand. Both differences are statistically significant with a *P*-value of 0.04. What will be the conclusion? An appropriate conclusion requires a clinical validation since 'statistically significant' is not synonymous with 'clinically pertinent' [2].

Demonstrable and repeatable

The Food and Drug Administration requires two concordant and appropriately conducted trials to demonstrate the efficacy of a treatment. What is the impact of such a decision on the power of a trial? If the power of each trial is 0.80, the global power of the two trials will be 0.64. Thus, the probability of detecting a difference is close to two thirds. If the expected global power for the two trials was 0.80, then the power to retain for each trial would be 0.90 [3].

Number of subjects required and feasibility

A working example will be borrowed from Hunsicker [4]. What is the number of subjects required for detecting a clinically relevant improvement in 1-year survival rate in renal transplantation? The hypotheses were based on the UNOS data. One-year survival rate was 84% at that time. For a risk reduction of 50%, given $\alpha=0.05$, $\beta=0.80$ and a two-sided test, without interim analyses, the number of subjects required was 560.

Now for improving long-term survival, let us focus on a risk reduction of 30%. The annual graft loss declines linearly after the first year by 6.9%, meaning that the annual rate would diminish from 6.9% to 4.9%. Assuming an accrual rate of 3 years and a follow-up of 2 years after the last inclusion, without interim analyses, given $\alpha=0.05$, $\beta=0.80$ and a two-sided test, the number of subjects required was 1500.

These examples show the difficulty encountered in renal transplantation in detecting an improvement in graft survival rate. The matter is even more complex today since mycophenolate mofetil (MMF) already improves the occurrence of acute rejection. In a recent study [5], an MMF-treated group (2 g) showed a reduced incidence (19.8% versus 40.8% for the reference group), and a reduced severity of rejection episodes. Better graft function was noted over 12 months, although graft survival at 1 year was similar (90.4% versus 87.6%). Thus increasing the intensity of immunosuppression appeared to reduce the incidence of acute rejection episodes but did not seem to modify graft survival.

The expected difference between a new treatment and a standard treatment should be even lower today than it was 5 years ago, and the number of subjects required even greater. New approaches are then necessary. The selection of patients and the choice of appropriate endpoints are important features in the design of randomized controlled trials. Let us explore two axes: reducing variation while improving definitions of enrolment criteria and concluding earlier with the use of surrogate endpoints.

To reduce variation

A matter of definitions

Improvement of quality and validity of clinical trials increases with standardized definitions of enrolment criteria and endpoints. Definitions of acute rejection for clinical trials would allow for standardized comparisons of outcomes. However, heterogeneous descriptions of the methodologies used to diagnose rejection and rejection reversal were reported in controlled trials [6]. An important effort has been made since 1995 to homogenize the criteria required to perform appropriate clinical trials in renal transplantation [6–12]. Standardized nomenclature of histological grading of transplant kidney biopsies has become a primary criterion for diagnosis of rejection in immuno-suppression clinical trials. International standardization in reporting of renal allograft pathology is useful for the design of clinical trials of new treatment strategies in renal transplantation [13].

A standardized classification of histopathology

A standardized classification of histopathology helps to define the inclusion and exclusion criteria. The Banff criteria allow the reporting and grading of histology at entry into a clinical trial. Patients can then be assigned to treatment groups according to their histological diagnosis, in particular in the case of acute renal allograft rejection. This is useful for defining new criteria of judgement, whether composite or not, searching for surrogate endpoints, exploring the prognostic value of histological parameters, refining calculation of the number of subjects required, selecting the variables to retain in a statistical analysis, and specifying the nature of adjustment variables. It also enables to study inter-center reproducibility of histological interpretation [12].

Qualification and quantification

The principal lesions indicative of acute rejection were ascribed to intimal arteritis and tubulitis. Glomerular, interstitial, tubular, and vascular lesions of acute rejection and 'chronic rejection' were defined. Acute and/or chronic rejection was graded using a numerical coding for each biopsy, scored from 0 to 3+. Arteriolar hyalinosis was also scored. Thus, six main diagnostic categories were defined as normal, hyperacute rejection, borderline changes, acute rejection (grade I to III), chronic allograft nephropathy ('chronic rejection') (grade I to III), and other [13].

Technical recommendations are part of the definitions

Technical recommendations are part of the definitions to ensure proper interpretation. Biopsy specimens must be obtained before therapeutic intervention and handled by experienced technicians. A minimum of two cores of renal tissue is recommended to avoid underestimation of rejection grade. Seven or more glomeruli and at least a single artery are required for proper interpretation in the Banff classification. Examination of serial step sections through the tissue samples is necessary to identify focal lesions of toxicity and to score intimal arteritis and tubulitis. Post-treatment biopsies should be discussed in large, multicentre prospective trials to study post-rejection changes. It was also suggested to promote prospective examination of structure-function relationships and long-term outcomes following acute rejection [8, 12].

Clinical-pathological definitions

An international database of acute rejection established from 19 transplant centres was designed to define standardized inclusion and exclusion criteria and endpoint definitions. Data comprised patient demographic parameters, induction and maintenance immunosuppression therapies, rejection agents (drug, dose, duration), clinical signs (50% decrease in urine and fever), serum creatinine (nadir, at rejection, daily during anti-rejection therapy to day 15, and at months 1, 3, 6 and 12 after rejection date), histopathological findings, morbidity, recurrence of rejection and function at 1 year. A parallel was drawn between biopsy grading, clinical parameters of rejection and response to treatments [9, 10, 14].

Acute rejection was defined [10] as an immunological process resulting in a serum creatinine increase of ≥ 0.4 mg/dl, with or without clinical signs, and should include a biopsy confirmation standardized to the Banff criteria. Corticosteroid-resistant rejection was defined as a rejection episode in which a minimum of 250–1000 mg methylprednisolone administered as initial therapy failed to result in stabilization or reduction of the serum creatinine after 3 days of corticosteroid treatment. Successful response to therapy required a serum creatinine level ≥ 110% of the serum creatinine on the day of the rejection diagnosis and a return of the serum creatinine to or below the rejection creatinine level by 5 days of therapy with maintenance of this response for a minimum of 30 days.

Analysis of rejection severity confirmed that standardized classifications such as the Banff scheme provided a reliable means for stratifying patients at risk of treatment success or failure. Biopsy grading was correlated with clinical parameters of rejection and therapy response. These data supported the use of the Banff criteria in clinical trial designs [11]. Further implementations were proposed by the Cooperative Clinical Trials in Transplantation that evaluated the pathologic criteria used for acute renal allograft rejection. Three categories of acute rejection were defined [12].

Clinical correlates of chronic rejection

Chronic rejection is characterized clinically by a progressive decline in renal allograft function and histologically by non-specific interstitial fibrosis, glomerulosclerosis and fibrointimal proliferation of intrarenal arteries. Late allograft failure is mainly caused by chronic rejection. The pathogenesis and treatment of chronic rejection are still unknown. However a search for clinical correlates is expected to improve our knowledge. They can be grossly classified as immune or non-immune, based on alloantigen dependency [15].

Chronic rejection mediated by immune phenomena is illustrated by the degree of histocompatibility mismatch and by its association with acute rejection. However, not all acute rejection leads to chronic rejection and new immunosuppressive treatments that prevent acute rejection have not yet been proved to reduce the incidence and severity of chronic rejection.

Possible non-immune risk factors were proposed: donor source or age, cold ischaemia time, delayed graft function, size mismatch, donor age, donor and recipient gender, recipient race, hyperlipidemia, and hypertension [16]. Further work is needed to understand these clinical associations in order to define the role these variables might play in the design of clinical trials.

Is it possible to conclude sooner? Surrogate end-points

Is there a marker of efficacy that would make a trial cheaper or enable it to be concluded sooner? Physiological or biomedical outcomes are used in clinical trials. However they may not be adequately related to the clinical outcomes. Thus, CD4 counts in AIDS turned out to be a poor predictor of mortality [17, 18]. Serum cholesterol is not in itself a problem but it can be the cause of many problems. It may be a surrogate end-point if one measures its level rather than the problems it causes. A surrogate end-point is a marker that is chosen as an indicator of efficacy in lieu of the one of substantive interest [3]. As illustrated by Senn, the difference between a surrogate and a true end-point is like the difference between a cheque and cash: you can often get the cheque earlier but then, of course it may bounce [3].

Does knowledge of the surrogate value capture the knowledge of the true end-point? [19]. A surrogate is a marker correlated with the end-point of interest and this relationship is the same across treatments. However, the fact that a specific end-point is correlated with the end-point generally retained for a given type of trial ('renal death' for example) does not prove that it is adequate. It acts as a correlative rather than a causal marker, given the different ways treatments may operate. Moreover, the interpretation of measures of surrogacy remains unsolved. For example, derived variance estimates and confidence intervals for the proportion of treatment effect explained by a surrogate in a Cox regression model have been shown to be highly variable [20]. What is an adequate proportion of treatment effect explained for a valid surrogate? Would we expect to find a surrogate that would explain 100% of the treatment effect? The difficulty of defining surrogates is that we need to run trials before reaching the end-points that will avoid us having to run them [3].

In a population of 627 cadaveric kidney transplant recipients, among those who lost grafts due to chronic rejection, decreases in renal function of 30% and 60% preceded graft loss by a median of only 1.1 and 0.7 years, respectively [21]. It suggested that little would be gained in a clinical trial that would use a pre-determined reduction in renal function as a surrogate end-point.

Could histological changes be used as surrogate endpoints? At present, graft loss due to chronic rejection and graft failure from any cause are the most reliable endpoints. Unfortunately, large numbers of patients are needed to demonstrate clinically relevant therapeutic effects on these endpoints.

Finally, one must bear in mind the Cardiac Arrhythmia Suppression trial [22], which compared two antiarrhythmic drugs with a placebo. The benefits of suppressing arrhythmia were counterbalanced by a death rate that was three-fold higher than in the placebo group. This type of pitfall outlines that inter-pretation of surrogate measures is still required as well as a better understanding of the mechanisms of treatments.

Alternative strategies for limiting the number of patients included in the study

Patient selection

It would be possible to limit enrolment to patients who are at high risk of developing chronic rejection. Thus, selecting patients already having a decline in renal function may reduce the number of patients needed in a clinical trial. However, selecting patients with advanced disease might diminish the effectiveness of therapy. Focusing on a too specific target population limits the generalization of the results. Finally, to approach the number of patients needed for a clinical trial requires preliminary data concerning the expected magnitude of the treatment effect [21].

Efficacy is different from equivalence

There remains concern for the long-term adverse effects of cyclosporine (CsA), particularly with respect to renal function and blood pressure. A randomized controlled trial was set up to establish whether withdrawal of CsA would alter long-term outcome. Conversion from CsA to azathioprine 1 year after renal transplantation improved both blood pressure control and renal allograft function, and was not associated with significant adverse effects on long-term patient or graft survival [23]. It would be interesting to know the power of a test that would show a difference when comparing long-term graft survival. In this type of design concerning long-term survival, do we deal with efficacy or with equivalence? This discussion is important since the hypotheses are different and the number of subjects required far higher in an equivalence trial [24, 25].

Treatment effect and uncontrolled study

'Borderline changes' in the Banff scheme are used for biopsies which show changes insufficient for a label of mild acute rejection. The appropriate clinical management for this situation remains controversial. Thus, the clinical course and response to antirejection therapy of 24 patients with borderline changes were compared with those obtained from 14 patients with mild acute rejection [26]. Patients were classified according to their response to antirejection treat-ment. Complete response to antirejection therapy was seen in 15/24 patients with borderline change versus 12/14 with mild acute rejection therapy ($p = 0.25$). Notwithstanding the discussion of the limitation in the interpretation of the results attached to the retrospective context of the study, what would be the appropriate conclusion on a treatment effect given no control group was constituted? The hypothesis being tested is not obvious. Moreover, one must not misinterpret a non-significant effect as an indication that the treatment was not effective rather than as a failure to prove it was: 'absence of evidence is not evidence of absence' [27].

Monitoring clinical trials

Monitoring the delivered dose: pharmacodynamics and pharmacokinetics

Pharmacodynamic monitoring may provide an alternative approach to traditional drug level measurement [28]. Pharmacodynamic monitoring measures the biological response to a drug and provides a method for the optimization of drug dosing. The pharmacodynamic monitoring of CsA involves measurement of the activity of the enzyme calcineurin; MMF involves an inosine monophosphate dehydrogenase; azathioprine, the activity of thiopurine methyl transferase; rapamycin involves the measurement of a P70 S6 kinase activity within lymphocytes; methylprednisolone involves the measurement of the endogenous synthesis of cortisol by the suppression of the hypothalamic pituitary axis. Additional clinical trials relating pharmacokinetics and pharmacodynamic parameters to clinical response are necessary to ascertain which provides the best guide for dosing and for monitoring clinical trials.

Monitoring adverse effects

Chronic vascular rejection is a cause of long-term graft failure after renal transplantation. A double-blind placebo-controlled trial was dedicated to evaluate the effect of misoprostol (added to standard immunosuppressive therapy) on the outcome of chronic rejection [29]. After entry of 40 patients into the study, the inclusion of additional patients was terminated because of a high incidence of withdrawal due to adverse effects: such effects (mainly gastrointestinal complaints) occurred in 3 of 18 patients in the placebo group and in 11 of 22 patients in the misoprostol group ($p < 0.05$). This situation highlights the importance of closely monitoring clinical trials to detect unexpected effects as early as possible.

Monitoring both efficacy and toxicity responses

The evaluation of a new treatment addresses both efficacy and toxicity. General methods for studying bivariate response data have been studied. A procedure was designed to allow early termination due to efficacy results, toxicity results or both [30]. The method is based on modified marginal sequential analyses, accounting for bivariate correlated responses and multiple analyses over time. Theoretical aspects have been presented in the context of normally distributed responses with extensions to bivariate failure time data. This approach is worth developing since toxicity is an important concern in transplantation.

Intention-to-treat analysis

A multicentre double-blind randomized trial, with enrolment stratification based on standardized Banff grading, was conducted to compare thymoglobulin, a rabbit anti-human thymocyte globulin, with Atgam, a horse anti-human thymocyte globulin for the treatment of acute rejection after renal transplantation [31]. The primary end point was rejection reversal. Intention-to-treat analysis demonstrated that thymoglobulin had a higher rejection reversal rate than Atgam (88% versus 76%, $p = 0.027$). What is in fact the justification for intention-to-treat analysis?

Departures from protocol are observed in most clinical trials. The question is then to what extent and how to cope with these departures. Some patients do not follow the protocol, deliberately or otherwise. Patients do not take their treatment (non-compliers), patients receive the wrong treatment (i.e. the treatment which was not randomly assigned), patients are not in fact eligible or patients are lost to follow-up. In the intention-to-treat approach the analysis is performed according to the allocated group of randomization whatever changes occurred subsequently. In this approach, any information regarding outcome is considered. Efficacy is then measured whatever the level of compliance. Alternatively, a per protocol analysis restricts the analysis to patients that completed the trial as planned. The idea is that a treatment which is not taken cannot modify the outcome, and information obtained from non-compliers is then irrelevant. However, the measure of efficacy restricted to the group of compliers only may be biased since non-compliers may differ in number, in pre-treatment characteristics or in types of treatment allocated. Several models have been proposed for obtaining reliable measures of relative efficacy from trials including non-compliers [32] and analysis of non-compliance was recently reviewed [33].

New approaches in statistical analysis

Improvements in statistical approaches are necessary to stick to clinical reality. Advances are numerous. We will illustrate two of these: analysis of correlated failure times and dependent censoring.

Correlated failure times are involved when the times to graft failure following kidney transplantation are observed but patients are clustered in different transplant centres. A specific approach is then required. Duration time models may include correlated failure times, due to clustered data. When used for survival analyses, these random effects hierarchical models are called 'frailty models'. They were applied to transplantation [34].

Transplantation is often associated with the incidence of recurrent adverse clinical events. In clinical trials designed to investigate treatments for such conditions it is natural to make treatment comparisons on the basis of event occurrence. However, when there is a more serious, possibly related, event that terminates the occurrence of the recurrent events, dependent censoring arises. Modeling strategies were developed to express covariate effects on the recurrent event process that address the possible dependence between the recurrent and terminal events [35].

Meta-analysis in transplantation

To assess whether prostaglandin E1 analogs have a role in either reducing renal allograft rejection or improving renal function among transplant and non-transplant patients, a meta-analysis was performed [36]. Nineteen articles met the inclusion criteria. Data were extracted on the basis of the study design, the nature of the study subjects and the main type of treatment investigated. Among the transplant studies, the rate of acute renal graft rejection or renal dysfunction was calculated for each study and then pooled using a random effects model. Mean change in renal glomerular filtration rate was compared between prostaglandin E1 and controls among both transplant and non-transplant studies and then pooled using an inverse variance-weighted method. Among transplant populations prostaglandin E1 did not appear to preserve or improve renal function.

This example illustrates the increasing interest in meta-analysis for improving the decision-making process [37–40].

Economical studies

Randomized trials are designed to explore the effects of treatment. They provide a context that allows pharmaco-economic evaluations. In effect, the purchaser needs to know which patients actually require which treatments, at which costs and for what benefits. Additional methods are required to convert economical outcomes into patient benefits. Economic evaluations are dedicated to establish links between monetary costs and health outcomes to allow optimal choices among the wide range of treatments available. Different types of studies are available [41, 42]. Cost minimization analysis compares costs for identical outcomes. Cost consequence establishes the consequences and costs of treatments but leaves the synthesis to the decision maker. Cost effectiveness uses medical units such as life-years gained and costs them. Cost utility converts effects into utility measures. Cost benefit converts everything to monetary equivalents.

Clinical trials offer a framework to allow pharmaco-economic evaluation. It is reasonable to think that an appropriate decision on therapy should be completed by an evaluation of its cost. This requires defining the types of costs measured (direct or indirect), the treatments compared and the types of outcome measurements such as quality of life outcomes; QALY's (quality of life adjusted years) attempt to produce an operating tool from multidimensional data.

Acknowledgements

Mrs Cécile Villette and Mrs Caroline Goldfrad are warmly acknowledged for their contribution to prepare this manuscript.

References

1. Senn S. The work of the pharmaceutical statistician. In: Statistical Issues in Drug Development. Chichester: John Wiley & Sons; 1997: 55–65.
2. Freeman PR. The role of P-values in analysing trial results. Stat. Med. 1993; 12: 1443–1452.
3 . Senn S. The measurement of treatment effects. In: Statistical issues in drug development. Chichester: John Wiley & Sons; 1997: 111–125.
4. Hunsicker LG. Design of trials of method to reduce late renal allograft loss: the price of success. Kidney Int. 1995; 48: S120–S123.
5. Halloran P, Mathew T, Tomlanovich S, Groth C, Hooftman L, Barker C. Mycophenolate mofetil in renal allograft recipients: a pooled efficacy analysis of three randomized, double-blind, clinical studies in prevention of rejection. The International Mycophenolate Mofetil Renal Transplant Study Groups. Transplantation. 1997; 15: 39–47.
6. Guttmann RD, Soulillou JP. Definitions of acute rejection and controlled clinical trials in the medical literature. Am. J. Kidney Dis. 1998; 31: S3–S6.
7. Guttmann RD. Acute kidney rejection: is there a consensus? Adv. Nephrol. Necker Hosp. 1997; 26: 165–170.
8. Gaber LW. Role of renal allograft biopsy in multicenter clinical trials in transplantation. Am. J. Kidney Dis. 1998; 31: S19–S25.
9. Cantarovich D, Soulillou JP. Efficacy Endpoints Conference on Acute Rejection in Kidney Transplantation: review of the conference questionnaire. Am. J. Kidney Dis. 1998; 31: S26–S30.
10. Guttmann RD, Soulillou JP, Moore LW, First MR, Gaber AO, Pouletty P, Schroeder TJ. Proposed consensus for definitions and endpoints for clinical trials of acute kidney transplant rejection. Am. J. Kidney Dis. 1998; 31: S40–S46.
11. Gaber LW, Moore LW, Gaber AO et al. Utility of standardized histological classification in the management of acute rejection. 1995 Efficacy Endpoints Conference. Transplantation. 1998; 65: 376–380 (erratum appears in Transplantation. 1998; 66: 1121).
12. Colvin RB, Cohen AH, Saiontz C et al. Evaluation of pathologic criteria for acute renal

allograft rejection: reproducibility, sensitivity, and clinical correlation. J. Am. Soc. Nephrol. 1997; 8: 1930–1941.

13. Solez K, Axelsen RA, Benediktsson H et al. International standardization of criteria for the histologic diagnosis of renal allograft rejection: the Banff working classification of kidney transplant pathology. Kidney Int. 1993; 44: 411–422.

14. Schroeder TJ, Moore LW. Efficacy endpoints conference on acute rejection in kidney transplantation: summary report of the data base. Am. J. Kidney Dis. 1998; 31: S31–S39.

15. Kasiske BL. Clinical correlates to chronic renal allograft rejection. Kidney Int. Suppl. 1997; 63: S71–S74.

16. Chertow GM, Brenner BM, Mackenzie HS, Milford EL. Non-immunologic predictors of chronic renal allograft failure: data from the United Network of Organ Sharing. Kidney Int. Suppl. 1995; 52: S48–S51.

17. Fleming TR, DeMets DL. Surrogate end points in clinical trials: are we being misled? Ann. Intern. Med. 1996; 125: 605–613.

18. Albert JM, Ioannidis JPA, Reichelderfer P et al. Statistical issues for HIV surrogate endpoints: point/counterpoint. Stat. Med. 1998; 17: 2435–2462.

19. Prentice RL. Surrogate endpoints in clinical trials: definition and operational criteria. Stat. Med. 1989; 8: 431–440.

20. Lin DY, Fleming TR, DeGruttola V. Estimating the proportion of treatment effect explained by a surrogate marker. Stat. Med. 1997; 16: 901–910.

21. Kasiske BL, Massy ZA, Guijarro C, Ma JZ. Chronic renal allograft rejection and clinical trial design. Kidney Int. 1995; 52: S116–S119.

22. Fleming T. Surrogate endpoints in clinical trials. Drug Inf. J. 1996; 30: 545–551.

23. MacPhee IA, Bradley JA, Briggs JD et al. Long-term outcome of a prospective randomized trial of conversion from cyclosporine to azathioprine treatment one year after renal transplantation. Transplantation. 1998; 66: 1186–1192.

24. Senn SJ. Inherent problems with active control equivalence studies. Stat. Med. 1993; 12: 2367–2375.

25. Jones B, Jarvis P, Lewis JA, Ebbutt AF. Trials to assess equivalence: the importance of rigourous methods. BMJ. 1996; 313: 36–39.

26. Saad R, Gritsch HA, Shapiro R et al. Clinical significance of renal allograft biopsies with 'borderline changes' as defined in the Banff schema. Transplantation. 1997; 64: 992–995.

27. Altman D, Bland M. Absence of evidence is not evidence of absence. BMJ. 1995; 311: 485.

28. Yatscoff RW, Aspeslet LJ. The monitoring of immunosuppressive drugs: a pharmacodynamic approach. Ther. Drug Monit. 1998; 20: 459–463.

29. Hilbrands LB, Rischen-Vos J, Hene R, Weimar W, Assmann K, Hoitsma AJ. Randomized trial of misoprostol in patients with chronic renal transplant rejection. Transplant. Int. 1996; 9: S41–S44.

30. Cook RJ, Farewell VT. Guidelines for monitoring efficacy and toxicity responses in clinical trials. Biometrics. 1994; 50: 1146–1152.

31. Gaber AO, First MR, Tesi RJ et al. Results of the double-blind, randomized, multicenter, phase III clinical trial of thymoglobulin versus Atgam in the treatment of acute graft rejection episodes after renal transplantation. Transplantation. 1998; 66: 29–37.

32. Armitage P. Attitudes in clinical trials. Stat. Med. 1998; 17: 2675–2683.

33. Goetghebeur E, Van Houwelingen H (eds). Proceedings of symposium on analyzing non-compliance in clinical trials. Stat. Med. 1998; 17: 247–389.

34. Morris C, Christiansen C. Fitting Weibull duration models with random effects. Lifetime Data Anal. 1995; 1: 347–359.

35. Cook RJ, Lawless JF. Marginal analysis of recurrent events and a terminating event. Stat. Med. 1997; 16: 911–924.

36. Ray JG. Prostaglandin E1 analogs do not improve renal function among either transplant or nontransplant patients: no further trials required. Transplantation. 1998; 66: 476–483.

37. Chalmers I. The Cochrane Collaboration: preparing, maintaining, and disseminating

systematic reviews of the effect of healthcare. Ann. NY Acad. Sci. 1993; 703: 156–165.

38. Petitti D. Meta-analysis, Decision Analysis and Cost-Effectiveness Analysis. Oxford: Oxford University Press; 1994.
39. Cucherat M. Méta-analyse des Essais Thérapeutiques. Evaluation et Statistiques. Paris: Masson; 1997.
40. Parmar MKB, Torri V, Stewart L. Extracting summary statistics to perform meta-analyses of the published literature for survival endpoints. Stat. Med. 1998; 17: 2815–2834.
41. Senn S. Pharmaco-economics and portfolio management. In: Statistical Issues in Drug Development. Chichester: John Wiley & Sons; 1997; 353–376.
42. Torrance G. Current experience with guidelines for economic evaluation in Canada. Drug Inform. J. 1996; 30: 507–511.

PART TWO

Is acute rejection an appropriate surrogate marker?

5. Surrogate end-points for clinical trials in renal transplantation

B. L. KASISKE

Introduction

Clinical trials are carried out to develop therapies that are best for our patients. Most clinicians would agree that the best therapies are those that have the greatest efficacy and the least toxicity, i.e. those that have the highest benefit-to-risk ratios. End-points in clinical trials are clearly defined events or measurements that reflect the efficacy and/or toxicity of therapy; they generally need to be understandable and reproducible and must occur frequently enough to allow therapy to be tested in a reasonably small number of patients over a relatively short period of time to make a clinical trial feasible.

The results of very early attempts at renal transplantation in non-identical twins were so uniformly poor without the use of immunosuppression that any improvement in graft survival provided convincing evidence of treatment efficacy. Indeed, so convincing were the improved results of transplantation in the early 1960s, using corticosteroids and azathioprine, that any randomized controlled trial demonstrating the efficacy of these agents in renal transplantation quickly became unethical and obsolete. However, the success with prednisone and azathioprine, subsequently enhanced by the use of antilymphocyte antibodies, set a treatment standard that necessitated controlled, clinical trials to prove that other therapies were more efficacious. The number of patients needed to conduct these trials, using graft survival as an end-point, was relatively large. For example, the Canadian Multicenter Transplant Study Group trial enrolled 291 recipients and found a significant improvement in graft survival with cyclosporine A at 3 years (69% versus 58%, $p = 0.05$) [1]. The European Multicenter Trial Group enrolled 232 patients and found a statistically significant improved rate of graft survival at one year with cyclosporine A (72% versus 52%, $p = 0.001$) [2].

Currently, short-term patient and graft survival rates have improved to such an extent that very large numbers of patients now need to be followed for prolonged periods of time to demonstrate that a new, prophylactic, immunosuppressive therapy improves patient and graft survival. This conundrum has investigators and regulatory officials searching for alternatives. One strategy is to develop surrogate end-points. A surrogate end-point is one that can be used in place of another for hypothesis testing in clinical trials. The purpose of a

P. Cochat et al. (eds.), Immunosuppression under Trial, 41–51
©1999 Kluwer Academic Publishers.

surrogate end-point is to reduce the number of patients, and/or the length of follow-up needed to test an hypothesis. For example, whether or not there is a complete and prolonged remission from a malignant tumor might be used as a surrogate for whether or not there has been a 'cure', or permanent remission. Having accepted such an end-point as a surrogate, clinical trials may need only to show that therapy induces a statistically significant improvement in the number of prolonged remissions compared with controls. The trial may not need to show that the therapy reduces mortality, although the implication is that it will. The number of patients and the length of follow-up needed to test whether a therapy affects the rate of remission may be substantially less than that needed to test whether a therapy affects mortality. Whether a similar strategy can be applied to clinical trials in renal transplantation is unclear.

The ideal end-point for clinical trials in renal transplantation

Clinical trials in renal transplant recipients can address conditions and end-points that are not unique to transplantation, e.g. hypertension and hyperlipidemia. However, clinical trials to test therapies that are essential for the success of renal transplantation per se are those that are directed toward improving graft survival and/or reducing complications of immunosuppression. Traditionally the most important clinical trial end-point in renal transplantation has been graft survival. Graft survival has usually been equated to patient survival with a functioning graft, so that failures are either loss of the graft due to rejection (or other causes of renal dysfunction) or loss of the functioning graft due to death.

It can be argued that deaths with a functioning graft should be excluded, or censored from an analysis of graft survival. Indeed, Matas and co-workers showed that kidney recipients who died with a functioning graft generally had good graft function at the time of death [3]. Deaths may be unrelated to the transplant, e.g. deaths due to automobile accidents. On the other hand, deaths may very well be directly or indirectly related to immunosuppression. Not surprisingly, deaths are more common in the elderly and among diabetics [4]. For testing the efficacy and toxicity of immunosuppression it is logical to combine these two separate causes of graft failure into a single end-point, since reducing graft loss to rejection is arguably the most important measure of efficacy, while losing a graft due to premature death may be an important indication of cumulative toxicity. Simply stated, death-censored graft loss could be reduced to zero by increasing the immunosuppression to such a high level that all patients die of its complications! On the other hand, combining the two end-points may obscure important information, since the pathogenesis and prevention of allograft rejection may be quite different from the causes and prevention of premature death. The best solution is to probably use two primary end-points, e.g. graft failure (which includes death with a functioning graft) and death, or death-censored graft failure and death.

Is acute rejection a useful surrogate end-point?

Acute rejection is attractive as an end-point for clinical trials testing prophylactic immunosuppression for a number of reasons (Table 1). Acute rejection episodes are still relatively frequent, and most occur early after transplantation. This reduces the number of patients and the length of follow-up needed for clinical trials to test strategies to prevent acute rejection. Acute rejection is also relatively easy to define [5, 6]. In addition, acute rejection and its treatment are associated with additional cost, major inconvenience and substantial morbidity, so that preventing acute rejection is beneficial. On the other hand, therapies that decrease the incidence of acute rejection may also have adverse effects that may occur much later, and additional end-points and longer follow-up may be needed to determine the benefit-risk ratio of therapy designed to prevent acute rejection. Although acute rejection may be an important end-point on its own, whether or not it can be used as a surrogate end-point for graft survival is less clear. Certainly, acute rejection would be a more compelling end-point if it could be shown that it reliably predicts subsequent graft failure. However, there are a number of reasons why therapies that prevent acute rejection, may not improve graft survival (Table 2).

The observation that preventing acute rejections may not always improve graft survival is supported by the experience of recent clinical trials. For example, three well-designed, randomized, controlled trials recently tested the efficacy mycophenolate mofetil (MMF) in preventing early acute rejection episodes. The results of these trials were pooled to increase the statistical power of the analysis [7]. In the pooled analysis, 1493 patients were included,

Table 1.   The pros and cons of acute rejection as an end-point for clinical trials in renal transplantation

Pros	Cons
Many predict graft failure	Many do not predict graft failure
They are common (increases power)	They are diminishing ($< 20\%$ in 1st 6 months)
Treatment causes morbidity/mortality	Prevention causes morbidity/mortality
Most occur early after transplantation	
They are easy to define	

Table 2.   Four reasons why effective prevention of acute rejection may not improve renal allograft survival

Not all acute rejection episodes cause graft failure, and those that do not cause graft failure are the ones most easily treated and prevented.

Therapies that prevent acute rejection may have long-term, immune and nonimmune toxicities that cause death with a functioning graft.

The second most common cause of graft failure (allograft nephropathy) may be unaffected by therapies that prevent acute rejection.

Therapies preventing acute rejection may cause renal damage that contributes to allograft nephropathy and results in late graft failure.

and the primary efficacy end-point was biopsy-proven rejection or treatment failure at 6 months. MMF significantly reduced the incidence of acute rejection from 40.8% for placebo or azathioprine controls to 19.8% for MMF 2 g/day and 16.5% for MMF 3 g/day. Nevertheless, graft survival at 1 year was not significantly different between the three groups: 87.6% versus 90.4% and 89.2%, respectively [7]. The results from a subset of 503 patients with 3 years of follow-up again showed no statistically significant difference in graft survival: 80.2% versus 81.9% and 84.6%, respectively [8]. Thus, although very long-term follow-up will be required to determine whether differences in graft survival may emerge, to date the 50% reduction in acute rejection episodes has failed to reduce the incidence of graft failure in these clinical trials.

That not all acute rejection episodes lead to graft failure has been clearly established [9, 10]. Rejection episodes which occur within the first few weeks after transplantation, for example, are not as predictive of subsequent graft failure as are rejection that occur later [11, 12]. It may be theoretically possible to select as an end-point a subset of acute rejection episodes that more reliably predict graft failure. For example, acute rejection episodes which occur late and are preceded by one or more other acute rejections are more likely to lead to graft failure [11, 12]. Some histological features of acute rejection also help to predict those which are more likely to lead to a poor outcome. For example, interstitial haemorrhage and findings of severe, acute vascular rejection have been shown to correlate with subsequent graft failure [13]. However, only a relatively small percentage of acute rejections have these histological findings and certainly not all of those patients have a uniformly poor outcome.

It is theoretically possible that some combination of histological and functional changes, with or without other clinical characteristics of acute rejection, could be used to distinguish acute rejection episodes that most often lead to graft failure. However, for several reasons it seems unlikely that histological and functional changes of severe rejection will be useful as an end-point for clinical trials. The number of severe, acute rejections is likely to be relatively small. In addition, since a relatively small number of patients have severe acute rejections, it follows that the majority of grafts fail without being preceded by a severe acute rejection episode. A well-defined, severe acute rejection end-point is, therefore, unlikely to be a useful surrogate of graft failure.

In general, the rationale for using acute rejection as a surrogate end-point in clinical trials has diminished as the frequency of acute rejection episodes has also declined. Prophylactic immunosuppression strategies that include newer agents such as MMF have reduced the incidence of acute rejection during the first 6 months post-transplant to less than 20% [7]. This information can be used to make sample size calculations for a hypothetical clinical trial that illustrate the effect of a reduction in the number of acute rejection episodes on the number patients needed. Let us assume that this clinical trial will use survival free of acute rejection during the first 6 months as an end-point (log-rank test for difference), and will compare a therapy to a control group treated with standard immunosuppression. Let us also assume equal randomization between the two groups, a two-tailed *p*-value of 0.05 and a power of 0.90. As the incidence of acute rejection episodes declines, the number of patients needed to show efficacy in reducing acute rejection increases (Table 3). Thus, the number of patients needed to conduct trials with acute rejection as the end-point is becoming prohibitively large.

Is the rate of decline in glomerular filtration rate a useful surrogate end-point?

A number of successful clinical trials in patients with renal insufficiency have used the rate of change in glomerular filtration rate (GFR) as a surrogate end-point for renal failure [14, 15]. These trials have measured GFR with plasma or urinary clearance techniques that require intravenous or subcutaneous injection of a marker, usually a radiocontrast agent such as iothalamate or iohexol. Disadvantages to this approach are largely ones of cost and inconvenience. In addition, there are a paucity of data in renal transplant recipients examining whether serial GFR determinations could be used to accurately measure changes in GFR over time, and whether such changes reliably predict patients who subsequently lose their grafts. Thus, it is difficult to conclude whether changes in GFR could be used as a surrogate end-point in clinical trials.

Serum creatinine is the most commonly used measure of renal allograft function. Changes in inverse serum creatinine should be directly proportional to changes in GFR, if other determinants of serum creatinine are constant over this period of time. Theoretically, this should make it possible to use changes in serum inverse creatinine as a marker for changes in graft function over time. However, few systematic studies have examined how well changes in serum creatinine predict graft failure. No major therapeutic intervention trials have attempted to use the rate of decline in GFR as a major end-point after renal transplantation.

A related approach to using the slope, or rate of change in renal function is to use a threshold change in renal function as a surrogate end-point. We investigated whether changes in inverse serum creatinine could be used as a surrogate for graft loss to chronic allograft nephropathy among 627 recipients of cadaveric renal transplants [16]. There were 122 (19.5%) who had lost their

Table 3. Sample size calculation for a hypothetical prophylaxis of acute rejection

Cumulative proportion rejecting in controls	Cumulative proportion rejecting with prophylaxis	Sample size needed ($p < 0.05$ and power 0.90)
0.40	0.20	266
0.20	0.10	702
0.20	0.15	2987

Assumptions: α (*p*-value) 0.05, power $(1-\beta)$ 0.90

graft to chronic nephropathy after a mean follow-up of 7.0 ± 4.2 years. Serum creatinine levels were measured in all patients at 6 months, 1 year, and then annually, thereafter. We first used a 30% decline in renal function (estimated by inverse creatinine) as a surrogate end-point. However, 60% of the patients who had a decline of 30% had not lost their grafts during a median follow-up of 3 years. The last creatinine clearance of those who had lost their grafts was still 50 ± 2 ml/min, suggesting that graft failure was not imminent in these patients. Thus, the number of false positives using a 30% decline in function as a surrogate for graft loss to chronic allograft nephropathy was relative high.

We next used a 60% decline in function as a surrogate for graft loss to chronic allograft nephropathy, and found that only 32% of patients had not lost their grafts after a median of 0.8 years of follow-up. Those who had not yet lost their grafts at the time of last follow-up had a creatinine clearance of 21 ± 2 ml/min, suggesting that most would soon lose their grafts. Thus, using a 60% decline in inverse creatinine as a surrogate was associated with very few false positives. However, the time to graft loss after a 60% decline in function was relatively short and called into question whether enough would be gained by using this surrogate, rather than waiting the additional median 0.8 year for graft failure. On the other hand, these calculations suggest that using a 60% decline in renal function as a surrogate could possibly shorten the length of follow-up needed (if graft loss were used as the end-point) by about one year. This estimation of the amount of time saved could be conservative, since serum creatinine was only measured annually. If creatinine had been measured more often, then the length of time to graft failure after a 60% reduction in renal function could be longer, and the time savings would be greater using this surrogate.

In summary, it may be possible to use serial measurements of renal function as a surrogate end-point for clinical intervention trials after renal transplantation. Either comparing the rate of change in function, or survival before reaching a threshold of reduced function, may allow studies to be carried out with fewer patients or shorter duration of follow-up than the same studies using graft failure as an end-point. Clearly, additional work in this area is warranted.

Can histological damage be used as a surrogate end-point?

As discussed above, some acute rejection episodes appear to lead to graft failure more often than others, and some histological features of acute rejection can predict a poor outcome. However, the relative infrequency of these findings associated with clinical acute rejection may limit their usefulness as a potential surrogate end-point. A more promising surrogate would be one based on histological changes from protocol biopsies, if such changes could be shown to reliably predict outcome.

Few protocol biopsy studies have examined how well chronic histological changes predict outcome. Isoniemi and co-workers obtained protocol biopsies on patients at 2 years post-transplant [17]. They defined a chronic allograft damage index which included the tubular, glomerular, vascular and interstitial changes that correlated best with decreased allograft function. Among 98 patients with 2 years of follow-up, the chronic allograft damage index was the best predictor of subsequent deterioration in graft function. In a multivariate, logistic regression analysis, individuals with moderately severe chronic allograft damage had a 3.75 times greater risk of deterioration compared to individuals with minimal chronic allograft damage. Individuals with more severe changes had more than a 10-fold increase in risk for functional deterioration [17].

Dimény and co-workers also reported that an increased chronic graft damage score in protocol biopsies at 6 months post-transplant was associated with subsequent graft loss at 3 years in 10 of 35 patients, while a low score was associated with graft loss in only two of 54 patients ($p = 0.002$) [18]. Others have reported that patients with chronic transplant nephropathy (Banff criteria) discovered on protocol biopsies at 3 months post-transplant (30 of 98 biopsies) had a lower actuarial graft survival (80.5%) compared to patients without chronic transplant nephropathy (94.4%, $p = 0.024$) after 58 ± 16 months of follow-up [19]. In future studies it will be important to establish the sensitivity and specificity of outcome prediction from such histological changes in independent patient populations. It will also be necessary to determine the reproducibility of the scoring by independent investigators. It is likely that more objective measurement of interstitial changes, for example using morphometric techniques, will be more reliable than subjective and semiquantitative scoring of tissue. Such techniques could substantially enhance the sensitivity of the technique for detecting patients at high risk for graft failure. Indeed, it is possible that morphometrically determined changes may be sensitive and specific enough to serve as a suitable surrogate for graft failure.

A recent study by Fioretto and co-workers illustrates the potential of morphometric techniques to increase the sensitivity of histological changes and thereby make such changes a more effective end-point in clinical trials [20]. These investigators compared changes in interstitial volume from native kidney biopsies taken before and 5 years after pancreas transplantation, to biopsies taken 5 years apart in a control group of diabetic patients who did not receive a pancreas transplant (and cyclosporine therapy). Although there was only a relatively small number of patients in both groups, they found statistically significant differences in morphometric measurements implicating cyclosporine as a cause of renal damage. This study illustrates the potential of morphometry to enhance the utility of renal histology as an end-point in clinical trials.

Alternative strategies that may reduce the need for surrogate end-points

The quest to define appropriate surrogate end-points has been engendered, at least in part, by a statistical conundrum. In clinical trials it is desirable to limit the number of end-points, so that the statistical power of the trial is not diluted by the need to account for the possibility that one or more of the results may occur by change, simply because several end-points are being examined. Trials are often designed to get around this problem by limiting the major results to one or two 'primary end-points', and at the same time analyzing the results of several other 'secondary end-points'. One possible corollary strategy uses a drug equivalency trial design. It may not be necessary to prove that each new therapy is superior to the current therapeutic standard. Rather, it may be sufficient to demonstrate that a new therapy is equivalent to the existing, standard therapy, with regard to primary end-points such as patient and graft survival. Having established the equivalence of a new therapy, with regard to major outcomes, it might then be possible that the new therapy has advantages reflected in one or more secondary end-points, e.g. cost or improved quality of life. Drug equivalency trials are designed to show that different therapies are equivalent, as determined by predetermined criteria, for one or two primary end-points. The number of patients needed in such a trial may be substantially less than the number needed in a trial designed to have enough statistical power to show a difference. Other differences between the treatments, e.g. cost and quality of life, can be explored in an analysis of several secondary end-points.

Equivalence trials are specifically designed to show that treatments have equivalent therapeutic effects [21, 22]. A range of equivalence is defined in advance so that any value in the range is considered clinically insignificant. If at the end of the trial the confidence interval for the difference lies within the predetermined range, then equivalence is implied. Equivalency trials may become increasingly important as therapeutic differences for major end-points such as patient and graft survival narrow. Demonstrating equivalency for these end-points may then allow investigators to focus on potentially important differences in one or more secondary end-points. A number of important secondary end-points are being used more often in clinical trials in renal transplantation.

Secondary end-points

Recently health-related quality of life is being recognized as an important end-point in clinical trials [23]. Although there is, as yet, no uniformly adopted method for measuring quality of life, various indices have been developed. In some instances a primary study end-point can be adjusted for quality of life, e.g. quality of life adjusted survival. More commonly, quality of life is treated as a secondary end-point. The use of quality of life as a secondary end-point has only recently been used in some clinical trials involving renal transplant recipients. For example, in a phase III multicenter trial comparing cyclosporine to tacrolimus, a number of quality of life parameters was measured [24], including the SF-36 and six other indices: current health, health outlook, health distress, Fleming self-esteem, Bergner physical appearance, and sexual functioning. The study concluded that transplantation was associated with significant improvements in quality of life, although patients treated for rejection had less improvement. In addition, there were significant differences between the two treatment groups in some health quality indices. It is likely that greater attention will be paid to health-related quality of life in future clinical trials.

A well-established risk factor is a close cousin to a surrogate end-point. The differences between a surrogate end-point and a risk factor is in the degree of outcome predictability. While a surrogate end-point is highly predictive of a particular outcome, a risk factor is less so. However, risk factors may often be appropriate, secondary end-points. Hypertension, for example is a well-established risk factor for cardiovascular disease which, in turn, is a leading cause of death after renal transplantation. It is probably not feasible to conduct a randomized controlled trial to prove that lowering blood pressure improves survival after renal transplantation. However, the evidence from general population studies that treating hypertension reduces morbidity and mortality is compelling, and there is every reason to believe that hypertension in renal transplant recipients is an important risk factor. Therefore, hypertension may be a reasonable, secondary end-point in clinical trials investigating immunosuppression or other therapeutic strategies. Similarly, other cardiovascular disease risk factors may often be suitable as secondary end-points.

Although it is neither a surrogate end-point nor a risk factor for disease, cost is an increasingly important secondary end-point for clinical trials in renal transplantation. Greater and greater constraints are being placed on health care resources. Medicine is reaching the point where expenditures for new therapies must replace those for others. As a result, it is important to demonstrate that a new therapy is not only efficacious, but is also cost effective.

Primary versus secondary intervention trials

Primary intervention trials are designed to test whether therapy effectively prevents disease. Secondary intervention trials are designed to test whether therapy is effective in treating disease that is already established. In renal transplantation, the distinction between primary prevention and secondary intervention may be more semantic than pathophysiological. This is due to the fact that it is often difficult to determine the onset of rejection. This is particularly true for 'chronic rejection' or chronic allograft nephropathy. For example, a population of patients who are high risk to lose their grafts could be defined by one or more criteria, such as decreased renal function or prior acute rejection. This population could then be randomly allocated to treatment or control. This type of hybrid between a primary and secondary intervention trial design could perhaps be exploited to enhance the power of clinical trials. Recent analysis has suggested that such a strategy could be effective [16, 25].

Summary

New approaches are needed for the design of clinical trials to test immunosuppression strategies in renal transplantation. The relative low rate of graft

Table 4.   Possible end-points for clinical trials in renal transplantation

Current/standard primary end-points
Patient survival
Graft survival that includes death with a functioning graft
Graft survival that censors death with a functioning graft
Possible surrogate primary end-points
Acute rejection defined with histological and functional changes
Survival before a threshold level decline in renal function
Rate of decline in renal function
Chronic histological changes
Possible secondary end-points
Quality of life
Cardiovascular disease risk factors
Risk factors for metabolic bone disease
Infections
Cancer
Cost

failure has meant that clinical trials using this end-point must be very large and/or must have very long follow-up time. Either of these requirements could have a very negative effect on future drug development. One strategy for dealing with this problem is to use end-points that reliably predict graft failure, i.e. surrogate end-points. For a number of reasons, it is unlikely that acute rejection will continue to be an effective surrogate for graft failure. Promising alternatives include end-points that measure changes in renal function or chronic changes in histology. Largely unexplored is the use of therapeutic equivalency trials. Proving equivalency for major end-points could be combined with hypothesis testing centered around several potentially important secondary end-points. This strategy may hold great promise for future clinical trials in renal transplantation.

References

1. The Canadian Multicentre Transplant Study Group. A randomized clinical trial of cyclosporine in cadaveric renal transplantation. N. Engl. J. Med. 1986; 314: 1219–1225
2. European Multicentre Trial Group. Cyclosporin in cadaveric renal transplantation: one-year follow-up of a multicentre trial. Lancet. 1983; 2: 986–998.
3. West M, Sutherland DER, Matas AJ. Kidney transplant recipients who die with functioning grafts. Serum creatinine level and cause of death. Transplantation. 96 A.D.; 62: 1029–1030.
4. Hirata M, Cho YW, Cecka JM et al. Patient death after renal transplantation – an analysis of its role in graft outcome Proposed consensus for definitions and end-points for clinical trials of acute kidney transplant rejection. Transplantation. 1996; 61: 1479–1483.
5. Guttmann RD, Soulillou JP, Moore LW et al. Proposed consensus for definitions and end-points for clinical trials of acute kidney transplant rejection. Am. J. Kidney Dis. 1998; 31 (Suppl 1): S40–S46.

6. Gaber LW, Moore LW, Gaber AO et al. Utility of standardized histological classification in the management of acute rejection. 1995 Efficacy End-points Conference. Transplantation. 1998; 65: 376–380.

7. Halloran P, Mathew T, Tomlanovich S, Groth C, Hooftman L, Barker C. Mycophenolate mofetil in renal allograft recipients. A pooled efficacy analysis of three randomized, double-blind, clinical studies in prevention of rejection. Transplantation. 1997; 63: 39–47.

8. Mathew TH. A blinded, long-term, randomized multicenter study of mycophenolate mofetil in cadaveric renal transplantation: results at three years. Tricontinental Mycophenolate Mofetil Renal Transplantation Study Group. Transplantation. 1998; 65: 1450–1454.

9. Braun WE, Popowniak KL, Nakamoto S, Gifford RWJ, Straffon RA. The fate of renal allografts functioning for a minimum of 20 years. Transplantation. 1995; 60: 784–790.

10. Peddi VR, Whiting J, Weiskittel PD, Alexander JW, First MR. Characteristics of long-term renal transplant survivors. Am. J. Kidney Dis. 1998; 32: 101–106.

11. Massy ZA, Guijarro C, Wiederkehr MR, Ma JZ, Kasiske BL. Chronic renal allograft rejection: immunologic and nonimmunologic risk factors. Kidney Int. 1996; 49: 518–524.

12. Matas AJ. Acute rejection is a major risk factor for chronic rejection. Transplant. Proc. 1998; 30: 766–1768.

13. Kasiske BL, Kalil RSN, Lee HS, Rao KV. Histopathologic findings associated with a chronic, progressive decline in renal allograft function. Kidney Int. 1991; 40: 514–524.

14. Lewis EJ, Hunsicker LG, Bain RP, Rohde RD. The effect of angiotensin-converting-enzyme inhibition on diabetic nephropathy. N. Engl. J. Med. 1993; 329: 1456–1462.

15. Klahr S. Levey AS, Beck GJ et al. The effects of dietary protein restriction and blood-pressure control in the progression of chronic renal disease. N.Engl. Med. 1994; 330: 877–884.

16. Kasiske BL, Massy ZA, Guijarro C, Ma JZ. Chronic renal allograft rejection and clinical trial design. Kidney Int. 1995; 48 (Suppl 52): S116–S119.

17. Isoniemi H, Nurminen M, Tikkanen M et al. Risk factors predicting chronic rejection of renal allograft. Transplantation. 1994; 57: 68–72.

18. Dimény E, Wahlberg J, Larsson E, Fellström B. Can histopathological findings in early renal allograft biopsies identify patients at risk for chronic vascular rejection? Clin. Transplant. 1995; 9: 79–84.

19. Serón D, Moreso F, Bover J et al. Early protocol renal allograft biopsies and graft outcome. Kidney Int. 1997; 51: 310–316.

20. Fioretto P, Steffes MW, Mihatsch MJ, Strøm EH, Sutherland DER, Mauer M. Cyclosporine associated lesions in native kidneys of diabetic pancreas transplant recipients. Kidney Int. 1995; 48: 489–495.

21. Ebbutt AF, Frith L. Practical issues in equivalence trials. Stat. Med. 1998; 17: 1691–1701.

22. Jones B, Jarvis P, Lewis JA, Ebbutt AF. Trials to assess equivalence: the importance of rigorous methods. BMJ. 1996; 313: 36–39.

23. Testa MA, Simonson DC. Assessment of quality-of-life outcomes. N. Engl. J. Med. 1996; 334: 835–840.

24. Shield CF III, McGrath MM, Goss TF. Assessment of health-related quality of life in kidney transplant patients receiving tacrolimus (FK506)-based versus cyclosporine-based immuno-suppression. FK506 Kidney Transplant Study Group. Transplantation. 1997; 64: 1738–1743.

25. Hunsicker LG, Bennett LE. Design of trials of methods to reduce late renal allograft loss: the price of success. Kidney Int. Suppl. 1995; 52: S120–S123.

6.   Is acute rejection an appropriate surrogate marker for clinical trials in liver transplantation?

O. FARGES

Acute rejection is considered as one of the main end-points in the evaluation of immunosuppressive protocols. The aim of this chapter is to assess the accuracy of this marker based on the particularities of liver transplantation.

How reliable is the diagnosis of acute rejection of liver allografts?

The liver is an organ which is easy to monitor:

1) serum bilirubin, alkaline phosphatase, GGT and transaminase are early serum markers of tissue injury and may be available within a few hours; these markers are monitored two or three times a day during the first week post-transplant;
2) Doppler ultrasound is a non-invasive procedure with which to explore both the vascular and biliary radicles that has a high accuracy and can be performed at the bedside;
3) percutaneous liver biopsies are simple and safe and are only contraindicated when there are severe hemostatic disorders (if such disorders are present, a surgical biopsy can be performed through a limited abdominal incision).

This simplicity is however misleading when it comes to the diagnosis of allograft rejection for the following reasons. First, impairment in liver function tests is not specific for acute rejection and may also be the result of graft damage (prolonged ischaemia, steatosis), technical complications (vascular or biliary obstruction), viral infection (CMV or hepatitis B or C reinfection), drug toxicity, or any systemic bacterial complications. Interpreting biological changes is extremely hazardous, especially during the first postoperative week. They are most likely due to anything else than an acute rejection episode. Second, although it was initially believed that Doppler ultrasound could help in the diagnosis of rejection, this is not the case. Finally, the typical histological picture of acute rejection of liver allografts is portal and central venous endothelial cell disruption, bile duct damage, and mononuclear cell infiltrate [1]. There seems to be good intra- and interobserver reliability in quantitation of these features [2]. This picture is probably specific for an immune response directed

P. Cochat et al. (eds.), Immunosuppression under Trial, 53–56
©1999 Kluwer Academic Publishers.

towards the donor antigen, but this immune response may be associated with either graft rejection or graft acceptance. In incompatible rat strain combinations where liver allografts are spontaneously accepted there is also histological evidence of rejection. The phenotype and in vitro function of graft infiltrating cells are qualitatively and quantitatively identical to that observed in rejected grafts [3]. The only difference seems to be in the T cell activation pathway [4] and/or in the progressive apoptosis of graft infiltrating cells [5].

Similarly, routine liver biopsies performed in liver transplant patients with normal liver function tests frequently disclose histological evidence of acute rejection that resolves spontaneously without any specific treatment [6]. As in the experimental model, this immune response is associated with an activation pathway against donor antigens which is distinct from that observed in patients with both histological signs of rejection and biological evidence of liver damage [7]. Patients with only histological signs of acute rejection seem, as in the rat model, to be protected against chronic rejection [8]. A histological picture of acute rejection can, therefore, be either a marker of graft rejection or of graft acceptance and cannot be interpreted and managed in its own.

What is the risk of misinterpreting a rejection episode after liver transplantation?

There still lack universal agreement on the definition of acute rejection which is considered, according to different centers as histological features of rejection, histological features of rejection with evidence of graft dysfunction, whether treated or not, or histological features of rejection with evidence of graft dysfunction that require active treatment. Hence, the reported incidence of acute rejection ranges between 24 and 80%. In fact, a more realistic interpretation is that approximately 20% of the patients do not appear to mount any immune response, 40% develop only histological signs of rejection, and 40% develop histological sign of rejection with simultaneous biological evidence of parenchymal damage. Only the latter should be considered as having acute clinical rejection, although it is currently impossible to ascertain that these biological changes are indeed related to rejection. Attempts to identify more subtle markers (such as soluble adhesion molecules) also prove inaccurate [9].

The second more pernicious (and less well documented) consequence is that whereas acute clinical rejection episodes obviously require additional immunosuppressive treatment, this treatment may have a deleterious impact in patients with only histological signs of rejection. There is indeed experimental evidence that immunosuppressive agents are also effective in inhibiting the spontaneous immune response leading to graft acceptance [10, 11].

What is the risk of an acute clinical rejection?

Early acute rejection episodes, whatever their severity, have no impact on patient or graft survival [12, 13]. Acute rejection episodes almost consistently resolve with increased immunosuppression and hardly ever result in liver failure. An early acute rejection episodes is (and is probably the only) independent risk factor for chronic rejection [14]. However, the incidence of chronic rejection after liver transplantation is less than 10% [14, 15]. In addition, chronic rejection may occur in the absence of a previous rejection episode, and it is possible that the immune response responsible for acute and chronic rejection are different [16, 17]. Chronic rejection may be treated by retransplantation with a risk comparable to that of a first transplantation, and patients retransplanted following chronic rejection do not appear to be at increased risk of chronic rejection.

What should the most appropriate marker be after liver transplantation?

Optimal management of liver transplant patients lies in the delicate balance between underimmunosuppression (associated with an increased risk of rejection) and overimmunosuppression (associated with an increased risk of sepsis and de novo malignancies). Rejection may therefore be used as an end-point, but only if the incidence of sepsis and de novo malignancies are simultaneously assessed.

Using the current immunosuppressive protocols, the proportion of death or retransplantation resulting from rejection or either death or de novo malignancies are comparable [14]. However, these proportions are unequal amongst patients and are influenced by the medical disease warranting transplantation and/or the immune status at the time of transplantation. An important objective is therefore not to consider transplant patients as an homogeneous population but to tailor immunosuppression according to indi vidual patient's risk.

There is increasing evidence that complete withdrawal from immunosuppressive therapy is possible after liver transplantation [18, 19]. Even if this is only possible in approximately 20% of the patients, the main objective is currently to reduce immunosuppression as much as possible in the long term.

Conclusion

Immunosuppressive protocols are currently primarily designed to prevent the development of acute rejection. However, by doing so, these protocols potentially also prevent the development of graft acceptance.

Acute and chronic rejection are not the predominant cause of failure of liver transplantation and in some patients, the risk of death from sepsis or de novo malignancies is greater than the risk of rejection. Paradoxically, the most appropriate marker of the efficacy of immunosuppression should probably be the ability to wean the patient off immunosuppresssion in the long term.

References

1. Banff schema for grading liver allograft rejection: an international consensus document. Hepatology. 1997; 25: 658–663.
2. Demetris AJ, Belle SH, Hart J et al. Intraobserver and interobserver variation in the histopathological assessment of liver allograft rejection. The liver transplantation database investigators. Hepatology. 1991; 14: 751–755.
3. Farges O, Morris PJ, Dallman MJ. Spontaneous acceptance of liver allografts in the rat: analysis of the immune response. Transplantation. 1994; 57: 171–177
4. Farges O, Morris PJ, Dallman MJ. Spontaneous acceptance of rat liver allografts is associated with an early down regulation of intragraft interleukin-4 messenger RNA expression. Hepatology. 1995; 21: 767–775.
5. Sharliand A, Shastry S, Wang C et al. Kinetic of intragraft cytokine expression, cellular infiltration, and cell death in rejection of renal allografts compared with aceptance of liver allografts in a rat model. Transplantation. 1998; 65: 1370–1377.
6. Dousset B, Hubscher SG, Padbury RT et al. Acute liver allograft rejection – is treatment always necessary? Transplantation. 1993; 55: 529–534.
7. Farges O, Buffello D, Shi YM, Berth A, Bismuth H. Anti-donor antibody class switching after liver transplantation. Transplantation. 1995; 60: 296–300.
8. Farges O, Kalil AN, Sebagh M, Reynes M, Bismuth H. Low incidence of chronic rejection in patients experiencing histological acute rejection without simultaneous impairment in liver function tests. Transplant. Proc. 1995; 27: 1142–1144.
9. Navarro VJ, Silver D, Langnas AN, Markin RS, Friedman AL, Pober JS. A pilot study of soluble adhesion molecules as surrogate markers for acute liver allograft rejection. Transplantation. 1998; 65: 126–141.
10. Harding FA, McArthur JG, Gross JA, Raulet DH, Allison JP. CD-28 mediated signalling co-stimulates murine T cells and prevents induction of anergy in T-cell clones. Nature. 1992; 356: 607–609.
11. Farges O, Buffello D, Moufetier A, Bismuth H. Prolongation of cardiac allograft survival following intraportal injection of donor antigens is inhibited by cyclosporine A. Transplant. Proc. 1995; 24: 2251–2253.
12. Neuberger J, Adams DH. What is the significance of acute liver allograt rejection? J. Hepatol. 1998; 29: 143–150.
13. Wiesner RH, Demetris AJ, Belle SH et al. Acute hepatic allograft rejection: incidence, risk factors, and impact on outcome. Hepatology. 1998; 28: 638–645.
14. Farges O, Saliba F, Farhamant H, Bismuth A, Bismuth H. Incidence of rejection and infection after liver transplantation as a function of the primary disease: possible influence of alcohol and polyclonal immunoglobulins. Hepatology. 1996; 23: 240–248.
15. Dousset B, Conti F, Cherruau B, Louvel A, Soubrane O, Houssin D, Calmus Y. Is acute rejection deleterious to long-term liver allograft function? J. Hepatol. 1998; 29: 660–668.
16. Dubel L, Farges O, Sato Y, Bismuth H. Development of anti-tissue antibodies in the rat liver transplant model. Transplantation. 1998; 65: 1135–1137.
17. Dubel L, Farges O, Johanet C, Sebagh M, Bismuth H. High incidence of anti-tissue antibodies in patients with chronic rejection of liver allografts. Transplantation. 1998; 65: 1072–1075.
18. Mazariegos GV, Reyes J, Marino IR et al. Weaning of immunosuppression in liver transplant recipients. Transplantation. 1997; 63: 243–249.
19. Devlin J, Doherty D, Thomson L, Wong T, Donaldson PT, Portmann B, Williams R. Defining the outcome of immunosuppression withdrawal after liver transplantation. Hepatology. 1998; 27: 926–933.

7. The success of clinical immunosuppressive trials in heart transplantation: the early detection of acute rejection

M. ANTOINE

Introduction

The development of heart rejection is a result of immunological microvascular damage. The small blood vessels contain an increased number of mononuclear cells which may also be seen passing through the vessel walls in the myocardium. The infiltration is focal but progresses and increases in intensity. The development of more severe acute rejection is associated with interstitial edema and myocyte necrosis. The grading of cellular rejection has been standardized by Billingham (Table 1).

In clinical experience, acute rejection in heart transplantation is treated above grade 2 or with hemodynamic instability. The deal is to treat before any myocyte damage occurs: this will clinically mimic an infarct and cause a decrease in the ejection fraction.

Diagnosis of acute rejection

Radiography

Radiographic evidence of rejection consists of progressive cardiomegaly and increasing pulmonary edema. The appearance of a cardiomegaly is occasionally an exudate from the pericardium. This pericardial effusion should be considered suggestive of acute rejection until proved otherwise. These appearances cannot be awaited as a reliable diagnostic aid in the recognition of early rejection.

Table 1. Grading of cellular rejection

Grade	Description
0	No rejection
1A	Focal perivascular or interstitial infiltrate without myocyte damage
1B	Diffuse but sparse perivascular and/or interstitial infiltrate without myocyte damage
2	One focus only with aggressive infiltration and/or myocyte damage
3A	Multifocal aggressive infiltrates and/or myocyte damage
3B	Diffuse inflammatory process with myocyte damage
4	Diffuse aggressive polymorphous infiltrate+edema+haemorrhage+vasculitis, with necrosis

P. Cochat et al. (eds.), Immunosuppression under Trial, 57–59
©1999 Kluwer Academic Publishers.

Electrocardiographic methods

Several studies have suggested that a change in amplitude of QRS complex could be used: the QRS voltage reduction is due to interstitial edema. Even with a high-frequency signal-averaged ECG with electronic filtering, the sensitivity is 82% and the specificity 81%. Intramyocardial electrocardiograms are also used with an implanted pacemaker. The value of this approach must be confirmed by other investigators.

Echocardiographic methods

Microvascular damage may produce acute diastolic dysfunction resulting from the onset of restrictive physiology. The decrease in compliance and increase in left ventricular mass is due to the edema and myocyte damage. A diagnosis of acute rejection is made from Doppler indices of diastolic dysfunction. The decrease in the isovolumic relaxation time or the pressure half-time is determined by analysis of the Doppler mitral flow velocity curve. This non-invasive method is a good adjunct but the ability to detect rejection is occasionally limited by insufficient sensitivity, effect of image variability and inter-observer variability.

Radionuclide methods

Routine myocardial imaging agents such as ^{67}Ga and ^{99}TcPP are clearly not specific enough to detect rejection until myocardial perfusion is lost.

^{111}Indium antimyosin antibodies have limitations, including delay of scanning and diagnosis and the inability to repeat injections due to the long half-time of indium. Apoptosis, or programmed cell death, can be detected by the use of ^{99}Tc annexin-V. The binding of the antimyosin antibodies to dying myocytes occurs regardless of the etiology of myocyte injury.

Cytoimmunologic monitoring

Due to the use of antithymocyte globulin, the progressive rise in the white blood cell count or in the total lymphocyte count or in the T11 lymphocyte subset is not helpful for detecting acute rejection. The eosinophil count seems to show a good correlation with the presence of acute rejection. Numerous cytoimmunologic variables have been measured, including prolactin levels, troponin, cytokines (tumor necrosis factor alpha), cytokine receptors such as (IL-2μ) and components of MHC class I antigens (serum β-2 microglobulin).

These might predict rejection, but there are important limitations to this kind of monitoring. Modification of the results may be due to events occurring in the periphery and not in the graft, and the values are not reliable in the immediate post-operative period because of the effects of the preoperative illness, surgical trauma and ischemic injury.

Some prospective studies are attempting to establish relationship between plasma nitrates (breakdown product of NO) and acute rejection. Future methods for the non-invasive diagnosis of rejection must detect molecular events participating in T cell activation.

Conclusion

The diagnosis of acute rejection in heart transplantation must be made as soon as possible, when there is a very low level of lymphocytic infiltration. Procedures confirming myocyte necrosis are only of use when it is too late to treat and save the patient. Endomyocardial biopsy still remains the gold standard for the diagnosis of acute rejection, echocardiographic study is also very helpful. Further investigations are required to prove the efficacy of another technique for predicting acute rejection, and invasive endomycardial biopsy may then become unnecessary.

References

1. Emery R, Miller L. Handbook of Cardiac Transplantation. Philadelphia: Mosby; 1996.
2. Patterson A. Chest surgery. Clin. N. Am. 1993; 3: number 1.
3. Rose M. Immunology of Heart and Lung Transplantation. Edward Arnold; 1993.
4. Billingham ME. A working formulation for the standardization of the nomenclature in the diagnosis of heart and lung rejection: heart rejection study group. J. Heart Transplant. 1990; 9: 587–593.
5. Yousem SA. A working formulation for the standardization of nomenclature in the diagnosis of heart and lung rejection: Lung study group. J. Heart Lung Transplant. 1990; 9: 593–601.
6. Trull A. Association between blood eosinophil counts and acute cardiac and pulmonary allograft rejection. J. Heart Lung Transplant. 1998; 17: 517–524.
7. Dengler TJ. Elevated serum concentrations of cardiac troponin T in acute allograft rejection after human heart transplantation. J. Am. Coll. Cardiol. 1998; 32: 405–412.
8. Marie PY. Detection and prediction of acute heart transplant rejection: preliminary results on the clinical use of a 'black blood' magnetic resonance imaging sequence. Transplant. Proc. 1998; 30: 1933–1935.
9. Richartz BM. Usefulness of the Qtc interval in predicting acute allograft rejection. Thorac. Cardiovasc. Surg. 1998; 46: 217–221.
10. Vriens PW. The use of technecium Tc 99 annexin V for in vivo imaging of apoptosis during cardiac allograft rejection. J. Thorac. Cardiovasc. Surg. 1998; 116: 844–853.
11. Stinn JL. Interferon gamma secreting T-cell populations in rejecting murine cardiac allografts: assessment by flow cytometry. Am. J. Pathol. 1998; 153: 1383–1362.
12. Bourge R. Noninvasive rejection monitoring of cardiac transplants using high resolution intra-myocardial electrocardiograms: initial US multicenter experience. Pacing Clin. Electrophysiol. 1998; 21: 2338–2344
13. Suzuki J. Sensitive diagnosis of cardiac allograft rejection by detection of cytokine transcription in situ. Cardiovasc. Res. 1998; 40: 307–313.
14. Derumeaux G. Detection of acute rejection of heart transplantation by Doppler color imaging. Arch. Mal. Coeur Vaiss. 1998; 91: 1255–1262.
15. Vijay P. Donor cardiac troponin T: a marker to predict heart transplant rejection. Ann. Thorac. Surg. 1998; 66: 1934–1939.
16. Cooper D. The Transplantation and Replacement of Thoracic Organs. Dordrecht: Kluwer Academic Publishers; 1996.

Some prospective studies are attempting to establish a relationship between plasma insulin (in cyclosporin) and acute rejection. Further work before the intravenous administration of rejection ... must define adequate insulin concentration [ref] cyclosporin.

Conclusion

The diagnosis of acute rejection after transplantation needs to reach as many recipients when there is a need for determination ... naturalized, to optimize adequate dosage. In conclusion, the constant of calcium and sodium patients, exchange transplantology will provide the good standard for the diagnosis. In some cases further comprehensive studies in the very state of critical investigations in requesting these the adverse effects of immunosuppression therapy regimens, and immunosuppression that being may become unnecessary.

References

[references list — illegible]

PART THREE

Towards long-term end-points

8. Factors influencing long-term allograft survival

C. VAN BUREN

As the demand for solid organ transplants has continued to outgrow the available supply of cadaveric organs, increased attention has been focused upon the steady attrition of transplanted organs due to chronic rejection. The UNOS published half-life for cadaveric renal allografts is approximately 8.5 years, not significantly different from the 7.7 year half-life published for cadaveric renal allografts under azathioprine-prednisone immunosuppression. This steady loss of functioning cadaveric renal transplants has led some clinicians to state that this loss is inevitable, due to the inability of current immunosuppressive therapy to influence the immunobiologic processes leading to chronic rejection. These include low-level B-cell activation and expansion of TH_1 T-cell populations directed against donor antigens.

While undoubtedly there are some pharmacodynamic failures for current immunosuppressive regimens, these claims that newer immunosuppressants have been ineffective in preventing chronic rejection ignore evidence which contradicts this therapeutic nihilism. First, the variety of immunosuppressive strategies, both for induction and maintenance therapy, are nearly as numerous as transplantation programs. These protocols result in dramatic differences in long-term graft survival. In fact published data include 50% or longer prolongation of cadaveric renal allograft half-life at numerous renal transplant programs when compared to pooled national data.

Furthermore, a large multicenter retrospective analysis of cadaveric renal transplants managed by cyclosporine maintenance documented that late rejection episodes usually resulted in loss of the allograft or permanent impairment of the function of allograft. The analysis noted that many of the patients who suffered late rejection episodes had significantly lower daily cyclosporine doses compared with patients who maintained good graft function. These authors imply that protocols that rely on low doses of cyclosporine combined with azathioprine may be inferior for maintaining long term function of cadaveric renal allografts.

Much of the controversy in determining optimum maintenance immuno-suppression has focused upon concerns regarding long-term nephro-toxicity of cyclosporine. Myers noted that progressive deterioration of renal function and even end stage renal disease was a consequence of long term cyclosporine therapy in heart transplant recipients; these complications were not observed in

P. Cochat et al. (eds.), Immunosuppression under Trial, 63–65
©*1999 Kluwer Academic Publishers.*

long-term cardiac allograft recipients maintained with azathioprine. Lewis failed to document the same progressive deterioration in long term cardiac allograft recipients, suggesting that other factors in protocol management may influence long term nephrotoxicity. These include avoidance of antihypertensive agents such as nifedipine which affect cyclosporine metabolism and minimizing exposure to other potentially nephrotoxic agents which may be additive to cyclosporine in nephrotoxicity. In addition presence of covert renal artery stenosis or cholesterol embolic injury to the kidneys in these heart transplant recipients may invalidate using renal function data of cyclosporine heart transplant recipients to predict nephrotoxicity in other populations of allograft recipients who lack these risk factors.

The difficulty in balancing the risk of nephrotoxicity against inadequate immunosuppression is documented in the studies correlating cyclosporine bioavailability to incidence of rejection. By routinely measuring cyclosporine pharmacokinetics and tailoring the drug dose to the patient's demonstrated absorption of the drug. Maintenance immunosuppression has been individualized for renal transplant patients at the University of Texas at Houston. Those patients who demonstrate large intra-individual variability in cyclosporine absorption are much more likely to suffer from chronic rejection than those patients who predictably absorb the drug. If one factors in the known poor correlation of cyclosporine trough level with area under the curve (AUC) calculations of cyclosporine bioavailability and the penchant of some centers maintain patients on very low cyclosporine maintenance doses, there is little wonder that these protocol decisions influence the half-life of cadaveric renal allografts. By maintaining therapeutic cyclosporine AUC concentrations, the University of Texas has maintained significantly better long term graft survival despite using significantly higher doses of a nephrotoxic immunosuppressant.

The difficulty in determining optimum long term immunosuppression is complicated by the advent of new immunosuppressants which in experiment studies are additive or synergistic when combined with cyclosporine therapy. The enthusiasm over mycophenolate mofetil (MMF) to reduce rejection rates in clinical transplantation when combined with cyclosporine has been tempered by the lack of an influence on one year graft survival. Furthermore, the combination of MMF with cyclosporine did not permit steroid withdrawal without a significant risk of acute rejection. In contrast cyclosporine combined with rapamycin both decreased the incidence of rejection and improved one year graft survival. The projected half-life for one year graft survival of primary renal allograft recipients is over 2 decades, although the follow-up thus far is less than 5 years. If these results can be duplicated in the general practice of transplantation once this new immunosuppressant becomes clinically available, then perhaps one can begin to improve the imbalance between demand for transplants by decreasing the number of transplant recipients entering the pool of patients with end stage organ disease.

In summary, based upon the diversity of outcomes of established transplant programs, the protocol for maintenance immunosuppression can indeed influence the likelihood of chronic rejection as well as the length of long term allograft function. There are clearly less effective maintenance immuno-suppressive programs which result in graft survival that differs little from the prior azathioprine era. Based upon published data, cyclosporine nephrotoxicity seems less a threat for long term graft survival than late occurring acute rejection or chronic allograft rejection. Newer agents, such as rapamycin, may make a major impact in decreasing allograft loss due to chronic rejection.

PART FOUR

Can we minimize the long-term side effects?

9. Patients' appraisal of side effects in quality of life assessments of immunosuppressive regimens

P. MOONS, S. FAIRCHILD and S. DE GEEST

Introduction

Quality of life has emerged as an important outcome measure in health care over the past two decades, and is increasingly used to evaluate treatment options. Indeed, understanding the quality of life implications of a new treatment modality in addition to studying its effects in terms of incidence of complications and mortality rate provides a more sophisticated and balanced view of treatment effects. Quality of life data offer a more complete understanding of the benefit/burden ratio associated with medical treatments in terms of patients' physical, emotional/mental and social functioning.

Quality of life research has already made important contributions to the allocation of health care resources, in determining reimbursement policies, and in individual medical decision processes. For instance, the Health Care Financing Administration (USA) [1] extended Medicare coverage of recombinant human erythropoietin treatment in dialysis patients based upon its improvement of patient fatigue and other physical symptoms – an improvement clearly enhancing patient quality of life [2]. Quality of life research has also influenced individualized medical decisions. An example of how quality of life may affect individualized medical decision processes refers to the choice for using FK506 in treating adolescent transplant patients as this immunosuppressive drug has a more favourable cosmetic side effect profile than cyclosporine.

In an effort to better understand quality of life issues for transplant patients, this paper will clarify quality of life definitions; discuss methods of quantifying quality of life; address present quality of life research efforts in transplantations; and finally assess the side effects of immunosuppressive regimen in transplant patients within a quality of life framework.

Definition of quality of life

Although quality of life is increasingly assessed in research and clinical practice, no consensus exists concerning the definition or the measurement of this multidimensional concept. Quality of life can include a number of dimensions that refer to physical, psychological, mental, emotional, social, spiritual and

P. Cochat et al. (eds.), Immunosuppression under Trial, 69–80
©1999 Kluwer Academic Publishers.

vocational functioning [3, 4]. Though some of these dimensions may be relevant to understanding specific human responses to a particular treatment option (e.g. spiritual beliefs), they are not necessarily regarded as pertinent to medical and health service research.

Based on the WHO definition of health, defined as 'a state of complete physical, mental and social well-being and not merely absence of disease or infirmity' [5], health related quality of life is operationalized by assessing the domains of physical, mental/cognitive and social functioning. It is the health-related quality of life that is traditionally measured in clinical trials and medical research to evaluate the benefit/burden ratio of new treatment modalities.

Testa and Simonson's [6] conceptual scheme of the domain and variables involved in quality of life provides a useful framework in unraveling the different components of health-related quality of life (Figure 1). This model operationalizes health-related quality of life based on the physical, psychological and social domains of health. Each of these domains comprises an objective as well as a subjective dimension. The objective dimension reflects the health status of a patient based on an objective evaluation of his/her functioning. The subjective dimension reflects patients' perceptions of their physical, psychological and social functioning. Both dimensions are relevant in that they contribute to a better understanding of patients' overall health-related quality of life [6].

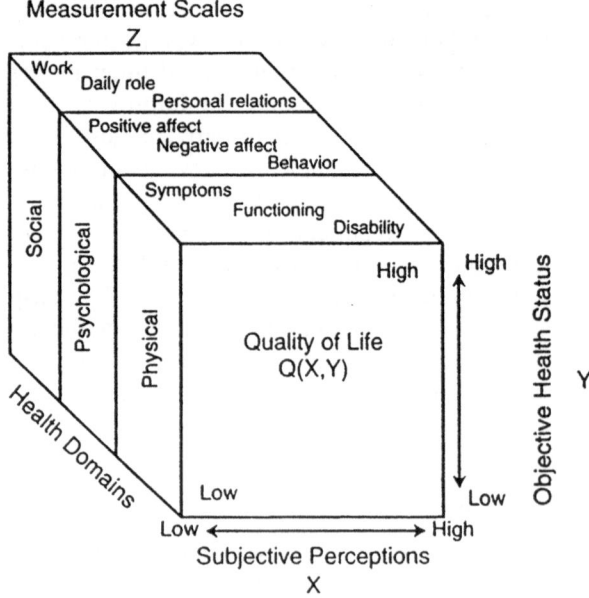

Fig. 1. Conceptual scheme of the domain and variables involved in quality of life assessment (from Testa MA, Simonson DC. Assessment of quality-of-life outcomes. N. Engl. J. Med. 1996; 334: 35–40. Copyright ©1996 Massachusetts Medical Society. All rights reserved.

Each of the three health domains can be further operationalized. For instance, the physical domain encompasses ambulation, mobility, fatigue, pain, sleep and ability to perform daily activities. Depression, anxiety, emotional well being and cognitive status fall within the mental/cognitive domain. The social domain of health-related quality of life includes work status, role functioning, personal relationships and sexual functioning [6, 7]. Again, each variable can be assessed from a subjective and an objective perspective.

Measurement of quality of life

Although quality of life can be measured as an unidimensional concept [7], a multidimensional approach in its assessment is preferred [6, 7]. A number of generic quality of life instruments have been developed to assess the different domains of health-related quality of life, including the SF-36, [8, 9] the Nottingham Health Profile, [10] and the Sickness Impact Profile [11]. These instruments allow comparisons among groups, but may not address quality of life issues specific to certain patient populations. In order to measure health-related quality of life of a particular patient group, relevant variables for each of the domains have to be selected and measured in an appropriate manner. Administrating disease-specific quality of life instruments allows a detailed evaluation of relevant quality of life domains for a distinct patient population, even though the possibility of comparison among patient groups is limited [3, 6, 7]. The merit of any study is determined by the overall consistency among the aim of the study, and the operationalization and the measurement of the concepts been studied. In other words, have the researchers selected reliable and valid instruments that adequately measure the appropriate quality of life domain for the target population? Because quality of life is a multidimensional construct, it must be measured as such. This has been accomplished by using both global measures of quality of life and disease-specific measures of quality of life.

Quality of life research in transplantation

The increased awareness of quality of life as a useful and meaningful parameter for clinical practice and research is reflected in an exponential growth of studies focusing on quality of life issues in the medical literature and more specifically in the transplant literature. Dew et al. [12] in their excellent quantitative analysis of the literature covering the time period between 1972 and 1996, found 218 publications addressing quality of life in organ transplant populations. These research studies include 14 750 patients, the majority of whom were kidney (46.6%), heart (19.2%) and liver (16.4%) transplant recipients. Bone marrow, pancreas/kidney, and lung/heart represented 13%, 3.1% and 2.7% of the subjects, respectively. Their analysis revealed that although transplantation does not restore quality of life to the level of healthy individuals, there is a clear improvement in quality of life from pre- to post-transplant in terms of physical functioning and overall quality of life perceptions. While the domains of mental health and social functioning also showed improvement from pre- to post-transplant in a number of studies, these results were not as conclusive as the physical functioning findings and the results on overall perceptions of quality of life [12].

Although Dew et al. [12] provide an extensive review of the state of the art of quality of life issues in organ transplant populations, we still know too little about specific immunosuppressive regimens, namely the side effects of immunosuppressive drugs and their impact on quality of life. This paper will now turn to the conceptualization and measurement of patients' perceptions of side effects associated with the immunosuppressive regimen and will discuss the findings of a study assessing renal transplant patients' symptom experience conducted at the University Hospitals of Leuven in Belgium.

Patients appraisal of side effects in quality of life assessments of immunosuppressive regimens

Life-long intake of immunosuppressive drugs is associated with a number of side effects that may have negative effects on morbidity and mortality, in addition to increasing psychological distress. Traditionally, side effects of immunosuppressive regimen have been evaluated based upon their impact on morbidity and mortality. Indeed, the occurrence of nephrotoxicity, hypertension, malignancies, osteoporosis and diabetes are closely monitored during the post-transplant course as they may negatively affect transplant recipients' clinical outcome. Going back to Testa and Simonson's quality of life model [6], health care workers have traditionally relied upon objective criteria as the primary means of evaluating treatment side effects. While the objective component of quality life has been well documented and integrated within clinical transplant practice [13–19], the subjective component is less understood.

Transplant patients' subjective appraisal of the occurrence of side effects and their perceived associated distress is a key to understanding the benefit/burden of treatment effects of immunosuppressive regimen after transplantation. Some side effects (e.g. impotence, muscle weakness, gingival hyperplasia) have little or no direct effect on morbidity and mortality, yet can be perceived as extremely disturbing by transplant patients. Assessing a transplant recipient's subjective symptom experience associated with his/her immunosuppressive regimen falls within the subjective domain of quality of life assessment.

Conceptualization of transplant patients' symptom experience

In order to define transplant patients' symptom experiences, concepts from the cancer symptom literature can be applied. Patient's symptom experience consists of two different although linked concepts: symptom occurrence and symptom distress [20]. Symptom occurrence, the cognitive component of symptom experience, can be measured along the dimensions of frequency, severity and duration of symptoms. Symptom distress refers to the mental anguish or suffering caused by the symptom and is the emotional component of symptom experience [20]. The following example illustrates the difference between symptom occurrence and symptom distress while also showing how these concepts are related. Male transplant patients can report increased hair growth, a side effect of cyclosporine; however, this may not be associated with increased psychological distress. In contrast, increased hair growth can be associated with major psychological distress in female transplant recipients due to the negative cosmetic effects. While both genders may cognitively perceive the presence of increased hair growth, the associated psychological distress may be different.

Relevance of transplant patients' symptom experience for transplant research and clinical management

For several reasons, transplant patients' symptom experience when measured by symptom occurrence and symptom distress is a relevant parameter for transplant research and clinical management. First, higher symptom distress results in lower perceived overall quality of life [6, 21–23]. Second, symptom distress may trigger non-compliance with the immunosuppressive regimen [24–27]. For instance a young female transplant recipient may stop taking immunosuppressive medications as the cosmetic side effects (i.e. changed facial and bodily appearance due to moon face, buffalo hump and increased hair growth) are extremely disturbing. Third, information concerning transplant patients' symptom experience can be used for pre- and post-transplant education in addition to giving patients information about the 'traditional' side effects of immunosuppressive drugs.

Measurement of transplant patients' symptom experience

Table 1 lists the studies that have assessed transplant patients' symptom experience associated with the immunosuppressive regimen. This has been studied in the renal, liver, and heart transplant population using different instruments. The first instrument developed in the early eighties was the Transplant Symptom Frequency and Symptom Distress Scale [21, 22]. This 27-item instrument measures symptom frequency (only one dimension of symptom occurrence) and symptom distress associated with side effects of triple therapy (cyclosporine, azathioprine and corticosteroids). Our research group performed consecutive adaptations of Lough's instrument [21, 22], which was used in three studies [28–30]. Recently, we revised this instrument into the Modified Transplant Symptom Occurrence and Symptom Distress Scale, based on a comprehensive literature review of side effects of immunosuppressive drugs, on our previous

Table 1. Studies on transplant patients' symptom experience associated with immunosuppressive regimen

Author	Year	Country	TX population	Sample size	Design	Immunosuppressive regimen[1]	Instrument[2]
Lough et al. [21,22]	1985/1987	USA	heart TX	n=75	Descriptive, cross-sectional	CsA, corti, aza or aza, corti	TSFSD
Foley et al. [38]	1989	USA	liver TX	n=26	Descriptive, cross-sectional	CsA, corti, aza	TSFSD
Jones et al. [23]	1990	Australia	heart TX	n=47	Descriptive, cross-sectional	CsA, corti, aza or aza, corti	TSFSD
Baumann et al. [39]	1992	USA	heart TX	n=29	Descriptive, longitudinal	CsA, corti, aza	TSFSD
De Geest et al. [28]	1995	Belgium	renal TX	n=148	Descriptive, cross-sectional	CsA, corti, aza	adapted TSFSD
Jalowiec et al. [31]	1997	USA	heart TX	n=173	Descriptive, longitudinal	CsA, corti, aza	HTSS
Moons et al. [29]	1998	Belgium	heart TX	n=105	Descriptive, cross-sectional	CsA, corti, aza	adapted TSFSD
Teixeira de Barros et al. [30]	1998	Portugal	renal TX	n=124	Descriptive, cross-sectional	CsA; corti, aza	adapted TSFSD

[1]CsA: cyclosporine A; corti: corticosteroids; aza: azathioprine

[2]TSFSD: Transplant Symptom Frequency and Symptom Distress Scale; HTSS: Heart Transplant Symptom Scale

research on transplant patients' symptom experience associated with these side effects [28–30], as well as by expert review.

Another instrument assessing transplant patients' symptom experience is the Heart Transplant Symptom Scale [31]. This instrument was developed in the late 1980s and assesses a wide range of symptoms related to heart transplantation. In addition to symptoms related to side effects of immunosuppressive drugs, this instrument also includes symptoms related to end-stage heart failure and symptoms related to complications after cardiac transplantation. However, this instrument only measures symptom distress, omitting the cognitive component of transplant patients' symptom experience.

In order to assess the subjective experience associated with side effects of the immunosuppressive regimen across different transplant populations, the use of the Modified Transplant Symptom Occurrence and Symptom Distress Scale is recommended. The use of this instrument will be illustrated by a study conducted in the renal transplant population at the University Hospitals of Leuven in Belgium.

Symptom occurrence and symptom distress in kidney transplant recipients

The purpose of this study was to assess renal transplant patients' symptom experience associated with immunosuppressive regimen. Symptom occurrence and symptom distress were measured using a descriptive, cross-sectional design in a convenience sample of 113 adult renal transplant recipients. Patients were at least 6 months post-transplant, Dutch speaking and literate. The immunosuppressive regimen consisted of cyclosporine, corticosteroids and azathioprine. The sample consisted of 70 males and 43 females with a median age of 47 years. Patients' median educational level was 12 years and median post-transplant status was 6 years. The majority of the patients lived in a stable relationship with their partner.

Symptom occurrence and symptom distress were measured with the Modified Transplant Symptom Occurrence and Symptom Distress Scale. This instrument identifies 29 symptoms related to side effects of immunosuppressive therapy. The items are then scored on a 5 point Likert scale ranging from 0 (never occurring) to 4 (always occurring) for symptom occurrence and from 0 (not at all distressing) to 4 (very much distressing) for symptom distress, respectively (Table 2). Validity and reliability of this instrument are discussed elsewhere [32]. Data collection took place during an outpatient clinic visit at the University Hospitals of Leuven, Belgium.

Research in transplant [29] and non-transplant populations [33–35] revealed that symptom experience differs between genders. Indeed, females generally report a higher level of symptom occurrence and distress. Moreover, genders also differ in the type of symptoms reported. A gender-specific evaluation of symptom experience is therefore indicated and this study accordingly performed separate analysis for males and females.

Table 2.   The Modified Transplant Symptom Occurrence and Distress Scale: example of item scoring

I have mood swings		The distress caused by mood swings is	
0	never	not distressing	very much
0	sometimes	at all	distressing
0	regularly		
0	almost always	0____1____2____3____4	
0	always		
I have muscle weakness		The distress caused by muscle weakness is	
0	none	not distressing	very much
0	a little	at all	distressing
0	mediocre		
0	much	0____1____2____3____4	
0	very much		

Since symptom occurrence and distress were measured at an ordinal level, ridit analysis was used to analyze ordinal data [36, 37]. A ridit represents the relative probability to an identified distribution. For each symptom of the Modified Transplant Symptom Occurrence and Symptom Distress Scale, a ridit was calculated for both male and female transplant recipients. The ridit was compared to the ridit of a reference group, which was achieved by summing the frequency distribution of the whole sample.[1] The ridit of a sample is the probability that a randomly selected person from that sample scores higher on the response variable than a randomly selected person from the reference group. For instance, given that the ridit for symptom distress for muscle weakness in female transplant patients is 0.617, a randomly selected female transplant patient will have a 61.7% chance of perceiving that symptom as more distressing than a randomly selected subject of the reference group (all transplant recipients in this sample). Ridit analysis has the advantage that data can be further analyzed parametrically, without violating the properties of ordinal level data [37].

Data analysis was performed at two levels, i.e. at the item level by calculating a ridit for each symptom of the instrument and at instrument level computing total scores by averaging the ridits calculated for each subject over all symptom occurrence and symptom distress items. For the calculation of symptom distress, those symptoms reported as never occurring on the symptom occurrence scale (score=0), were excluded from analysis, in order to avoid anticipatory symptom distress [29]. Level of significance was set at $p < 0.05$.

---

[1]E.g.: Frequency distribution for symptom occurrence of bruises: Male renal transplant patients: 0=14; 1=11; 2=12; 3=7; 4=6/Female renal transplant patients: 0=4; 1=10; 2=6; 3=3; 4=12. Reference group for bruises: 0=28; 1=21; 2=18; 3=10; 4=18

Results

The comparison of the symptom experience between males and females showed that female renal transplant patients experienced a significantly higher level of both symptom occurrence and symptom distress than did males (Figure 2) ($p < 0.0001$). A ridit of 0.57 for symptom distress indicates that an arbitrarily selected woman from this sample has a 57% chance of scoring higher on symptom distress than an arbitrarily selected patient from the whole sample. In contrast, an arbitrarily selected man has a 46% chance of scoring higher than an arbitrarily selected patient of the whole sample. In other words, the probability of a higher degree of symptom distress is higher in females than in males.

A rank order of the 10 most frequently occurring and distressing symptoms was made based on the symptom ridits of male and female renal transplant recipients, respectively (Tables 3 and 4). Symptoms such as bruises, increased hair growth, muscle weakness, fatigue, fragile skin, poor vision, increased appetite and decreased interest in sex occurred in both males and females both. Male recipients reported acne and tremor, while women had problems with sleeplessness and moon face.

The most distressing symptom in male and female transplant patients was impotence and muscle weakness, respectively. The list of the ten most distressing symptoms showed less concordance among genders compared to the list of symptom occurrence. Only muscle weakness, poor vision, and sleeplessness were perceived as disturbing by both genders. Based on the results it can be concluded that females are more distressed by externally visible symptoms than are men. Bruises, the most occurring symptom in male renal transplant recipients, seemed to cause little distress. This illustrates that the most occurring symptom is therefore not always the most distressing, and vice versa.

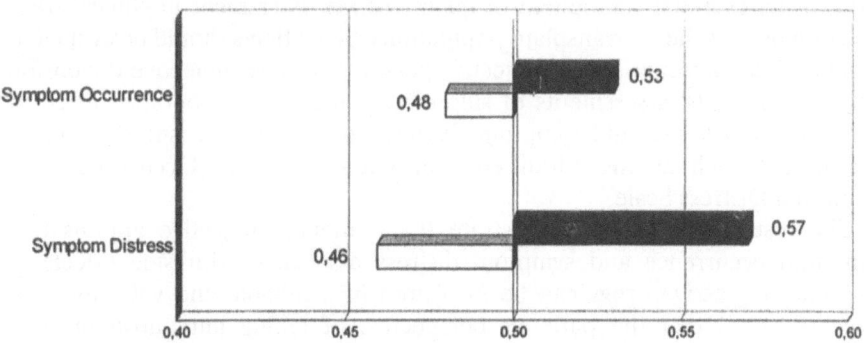

Fig. 2. Comparison of symptom experience between men (w) and women (W)

Table 3.   The 10 most frequent symptoms in male and female renal
transplant recipients

Men ($n=70$)	Women ($n=43$)
1. Bruises	1. Fragile skin
2. Increased hair growth	2. Bruises
3. Muscle weakness	3. Increased hair growth
4. Fatigue	4. Decreased interest in sex
5. Fragile skin	5. Muscle weakness
6. Poor vision	6. Increased appetite
7. Increased appetite	7. Sleeplessness
8. Acne	8. Fatigue
9. Decreased interest in sex	9. Poor vision
10. Tremor	10. Moon face

Table 4.   The 10 most distressing symptoms in male and female renal
transplant recipients

Men ($n=70$)	Women ($n=43$)
1. Impotence	1. Muscle weakness
2. Back pain	2. Headache
3. Poor vision	3. Gingival hyperplasia
4. Muscle weakness	4. Fragile skin
5. Stomach complaints	5. Increased hair growth
6. Sleeplessness	6. Fever
7. Skin rash	7. Sleeplessness
8. Decreased interest in sex	8. Bruises
9. Diarrhea	9. Poor vision
10. Muscle cramps	10. Swollen ankles

Conclusion

Quality of life is becoming an increasingly important parameter used to
evaluate treatment outcomes. Evaluation of side effects of immunosuppressive
drugs is an essential component of quality of life assessment in clinical trials
and outcome studies in transplant populations. Side effects should be evaluated
from both an objective and a subjective perspective. The subjective dimension
refers to patients' assessments of side effects and can be operationalized as
symptom occurrence and symptom distress and can be measured using an
instrument such as the Modified Transplant Symptom Occurrence and
Symptom Distress Scale.

The results of this study illustrate that patients' subjective appraisal of
symptom occurrence and symptom distress associated with side effects of
immunosuppressive drugs can be measured in a reliable and valid manner.
Results reveal that the patient's perspective of taking immunosuppressive
medications when assessed through symptom occurrence and symptom distress
is markedly different from the health care worker's perspective. In the past,
clinicians have traditionally focused on those side effects that may negatively

affect clinical outcomes during transplant patients' life long follow-up (i.e. nephrotoxicity, hypertension, cancer, osteoporosis and diabetes). Differences between genders in terms of symptom experience should guide transplant clinicians in a gender specific clinical management of side effects of immuno-suppressive drugs.

Data on symptom occurrence and symptom distress contributes to the development of a comprehensive symptomatological profile of immunosup-pressive regimens which is both objective and subjective. This duel approach to assessing quality of life will contribute to the state-of-the-art of transplant medicine.

References

1. Office of Technology Assessment. Recombinant Human Erythropoietin: Payment Options for Medicare. Publication No. OTA-H-451. Washington, DC: United States Government Printing Office, 1990.
2. Canadian Erythropoietin Study Group. Association between recombinant human erythro-poietin and quality of life and exercise capacity of patients receiving haemodialysis. BMJ. 1990; 300: 573–578.
3. Raeburn JM, Rootman I. Quality of life and health promotion. In: Renwick R, Brown I, Nagler M, editors. Quality of Life in Health Promotion and Rehabilitation. Thousand Oaks: Sage Publications; 1996: 14–25.
4. Felce D. Defining and applying the concept of quality of life. J. Intellect. Disabil. Res. 1997; 41: 126–135.
5. World Health Organization. Constitution in Basic Documents. Geneva: WHO, 1948.
6. Testa MA, Simonson DC. Assessment of quality-of-life outcomes. N. Engl. J. Med. 1996; 334: 35–40.
7. Dew MA, Regalski JM, Switzer GE, Allen AS. Quality of life in organ transplantation: Effects on adult recipients and their families. In: Trzepacz PT, DiMartini A, editors. Transplantation Psychiatry: Issues for the 90s. New York: Cambridge University Press, in press.
8. McHorney CA, Ware JE Jr, Lu JF, Sherbourne CD. The MOS 36-item Short-Form Health Survey (SF-36): III. Tests of data quality, scaling assumptions, and reliability across diverse patient groups. Med. Care. 1994; 32: 40–66.
9. Ware JE Jr, Sherbourne CD. The MOS 36-item short-form health survey (SF-36). I. Conceptual framework and item selection. Med. Care. 1992; 30: 473–483.
10. Hunt SM, McKenna SP, McEwen J, Williams J, Papp E. The Nottingham Health Profile: subjective health status and medical consultations. Soc. Sci. Med. 1981; 15: 221–229.
11. Bergner M, Bobbitt RA, Carter WB, Gilson BS. The Sickness Impact Profile: development and final revision of a health status measure. Med. Care. 1981; 19: 787–805.
12. Dew MA, Switzer GE, Goycoolea, JM et al: Does transplantation produce quality of life benefits? Transplantation. 1997; 64: 1261–1273.
13. Bernabeu M, Krupp P, Wiskott E. Long-term safety of cyclosporine in renal transplant reci-pients: worldwide experience. Transplant. Proc. 1993; 25: 17–19.
14. Graham RM. Cyclosporine: mechanisms of action and toxicity. Cleveland Clin. J. Med. 1994; 61: 308–313.
15. Kahan BD, Flechner SM, Lorber MI, Golden D, Conley S, Van Buren CT. Complications of cyclosporine-prednisone immunosuppression in 402 renal allograft recipients exclusively followed at a single center for from one to five years. Transplantation. 1987; 43: 197–204.
16. Morris-Stiff G, Ostrowski K, Balaji V et al. Prospective randomised study comparing tacro-limus (Prograf) and cyclosporin (Neoral) as primary immunosuppression in cadaveric renal

transplants at a single institution: interim report of the first 80 cases. Transplant. Int. 1998; 11: S334–S336.

17. Pasha TM, Wiesner RH, Dahlke LM, Porayko MK, Krom RAF. An open-label study of the safety and tolerability of converting stable liver transplant recipients to neoral. Liver. Transplant. Surg. 1998; 4: 410–415.

18. Seale JP, Compton MR. Side-effects of corticosteroid agents. Med. J. Aust. 1986; 144: 139–142.

19. Taylor DO. The use of tacrolimus and mycophenolate mofetil after cardiac transplantation. Curr. Opin. Cardiol. 1997; 12: 161–165.

20. Rhodes VA, Watson PM. Symptom distress, the concept: past and present. Semin. Oncol. 1987; 3: 242–247.

21. Lough ME, Lindsey AM, Shinn JA, Stotts NA. Life satisfaction following heart transplantation. J. Heart Transplant. 1985; 4: 446–449.

22. Lough ME, Lindsey AM, Shinn JA, Stotts NA. Impact of symptom frequency and symptom distress on self-reported quality of life in heart transplant recipients. Heart Lung. 1987; 16: 193–200.

23. Jones BM, Taylor FJ, Wright OM et al. Quality of life after heart transplantation in patients assigned to double- or triple-drug therapy. J. Heart Transplant. 1990; 9: 392–396.

24. De Geest S, Abraham I, Dunbar-Jacob J, Vanhaecke J. The significance of noncompliance in the etiology of acute late rejections in the heart transplant population. Circulation. 1997; 96: I-15.

25. Didlake RH, Dreyfus K, Kerman RH, Van Buren CT, Kahan BD. Patient non-compliance: a major cause of late graft failure in cyclosporine-treated renal transplants. Transplant. Proc. 1988; 10 (suppl.3): 63–69.

26. Schweitzer RT, Rovelli M, Palmeri D, Vossler E, Hull D, Bartus S. Non-compliance in organ transplant recipients. Transplantation. 1990; 49: 374–377.

27. Sketris I, Grobler M, West M, Gerus S. Factors affecting compliance with cyclosporine in adult renal transplant recipients. Transplant. Proc. 1994; 26: 2538–2541.

28. De Geest S, Borgermans L, Gemoets H et al. Incidence, determinants, and consequences of subclinical non-compliance with immunosuppressive therapy in renal transplant recipients. Transplantation. 1995; 59: 340–347.

29. Moons P, De Geest S, Abraham I, Van Cleemput J, Vanhaecke J. Symptom experience associated with maintenance immunosuppression after heart transplantation: patients' appraisal of side effects. Heart Lung. 1998; 27: 315–325.

30. Teixeira de Barros C, Cabrita J, Pena JR. Self-report of symptom frequency and symptom distress in kidney transplant recipients. In: Pharmacoepidemiology and Drug Safety. Abstract supplement; 1998 August 16–19; Berlin, Germany. New York: Wiley, 1998.

31. Jalowiec A, Grady KL, White-Williams C et al. Symptom distress three months after heart transplantation. J. Heart Lung. Transplant. 1997; 16: 604–614.

32. De Geest S, Moons P, Versteven K, Vlaminck H, Moens G, Waer M. Validity and reliability of the Modified Transplant Symptom Occurrence and Symptom Distress Scale. In: Transplant 98 Book of Abstracts; 1998 July 12–17; Montréal, Canada. The Transplantation Society, 1998.

33. Gijsbers van Wijk CM, Kolk AM, van den Bosch WJ, van den Hoogen HJ. Male and female morbidity in general practice: the nature of sex differences. Soc. Sci. Med. 1992; 35: 665–678.

34. Lieban RW. Gender and symptom sensitivity: report on a Philippine study. Am. J. Orthopsychiatry. 1985; 55: 446–450.

35. Verbrugge LM. Gender and health: an update on hypotheses and evidence. J. Health Soc. Behav. 1985; 26: 156–182.

36. Bross IDJ. How to use ridit analysis. Biometrics. 1958; 14: 18–38.

37. Sermeus W, Delesie L. Ridit analysis on ordinal data. West. J. Nurs. Res. 1996; 18: 351–359.

38. Foley TC, Davis CP, Conway PA. Liver transplant recipients – self-report of symptom frequency, symptom distress, quality of life. Transplant. Proc. 1989; 21: 2417–2418.

39. Baumann LJ, Young CJ, Egan JJ. Living with a heart transplant: long-term adjustment. Transplant. Int. 1992; 5: 1–8.

10. Cardiovascular complications after renal transplantation

V. SCHWENGER, M. ZEIER, M. WIESEL and E. RITZ

Epidemiology of cardiovascular death after transplantation

According to Lindholm [1] between the second and fifth year after renal transplantation, 41.4% of graft loss is accounted for by rejection and no less than 49.2% by death with a functioning graft, while other causes account for a further 9.4%. Thus, reduction of cardiovascular death will be a very efficient measure to preserve grafts. According to the EDTA Registry [2], the frequency of death from cardiovascular causes increases markedly with age in patients with a functioning graft who had suffered from standard primary renal disease. The recent summary on cardiovascular disease in renal patients by the National Kidney Foundation (Table 1) states that clinical coronary artery disease and left ventricular hypertrophy by echocardiography are definitely more frequent in recipients with renal grafts, although substantially less so than in patients on hemodialysis or peritoneal dialysis [3]. The survival advantage conferred by transplantation is well illustrated by the studies of Port et al. [4] and Bonal et al. [5]. The relative mortality of graft recipients beyond the first month after transplantation was substantially lower, particularly in diabetic patients [4] and high risk elderly patients [5], than in hemodialysed patients on the transplant waiting list. In the study of the Catalunya registry, cardiovascular comorbidity was also substantially lower in transplanted patients (Figure 1) and this was paralleled by substantially better actuarial 5-year survival (0.86 after transplantation versus 0.77 on hemodialysis). Using multivariate analysis Cosio [6] found that apart from age, diabetes and smoking, length of time on dialysis was an independent predictor of post-transplantation death. In contrast, duration of pretransplantation dialysis treatment was not an independent predictor in the study of Arend [7], but there is little doubt that much of the pathology causing cardiac death after transplantation has been acquired in the pretransplantation period of endstage renal failure. This is indicated by several studies [8, 9] which document that cardiovascular abnormalities at the time of transplantation are independent and potent predictors of subsequent death with functioning graft. In the study of MacGregor [8] left ventricular mass index (LVM) was significantly higher in those patients who subsequently died (median 167 versus 134 g/m^2, p 0.03) as were end-systolic (4.3 versus 3.4 cm, p 0.01) and end-diastolic (5.8 versus 5.2 cm. p <0.01) diameters and systolic

P. Cochat et al. (eds.), Immunosuppression under Trial, 81–88
©1999 Kluwer Academic Publishers.

Table 1.   Prevalence of cardiovascular problems in patients on renal replacement therapy (after ref. [3])

	Coronary disease (by clinical signs/symptoms)	Left ventricular hypertrophy (by echocardiography)
General population	5–(12)%	20%
Hemodialysis	40%	75%
Peritoneal dialysis	40%	75%
Renal transplantation	15%	50%

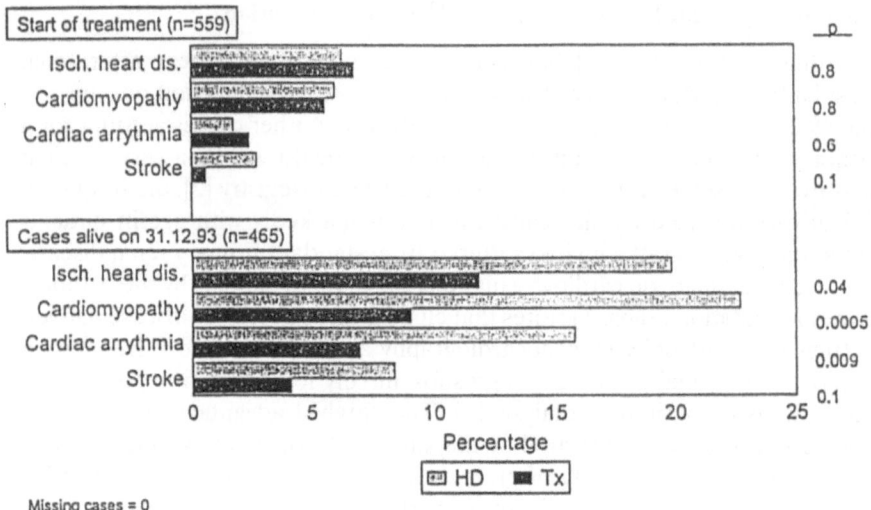

Missing cases = 0

Fig. 1.   Proportion of patients with cardiovascular comorbidity: comparison of elderly transplanted patients (TX) and hemodialysed patients (HD) on the waiting list (after [5]).

dysfunction (fractional shortening 27 versus 33, $p < 0.01$). Further studies are required to asses to what extent echocardiographic studies exaggerate the frequency of left ventricular hypertrophy (LVH) by artefactual overestimation of LVM when hypervolemia and cardiac dilatation are present. It has been claimed that in graft recipients LVH is more prominent in patients with the DD genotype of the ACE gene polymorphism [10]. In a prospective Canadian cohort study in which patients were followed with echocardiography, successful renal transplantation led to significant reversal of systolic dysfunction, concentric LVH and LV dilatation [11]. Of note, de novo ischemic heart disease developed only in one of 102 patients, in contrast to a recent follow-up study in which 23% of patients with a functioning graft for 15 years developed de novo coronary heart disease [12]. Apparently partial reversal of LVH [11] is incomplete. Cardiac pathology and risk of cardiac death are not normalized in this population and the remarkable rate of de novo development of coronary disease may play a role [12, 13].

Hypertension

Elevated blood pressure values or at least blood pressure values above those recommended by the Joint National Committee (JNC VI), i.e. 130/85 mmHg [14], are present in the great majority of patients after renal transplantation, particularly those treated with cyclosporin A. The factors involved in the genesis of hypertension have been reviewed recently [15] and a detailed discussion is beyond the scope of this analysis. Recent studies have shown [16] that blood pressure has a major impact on long-term graft outcome. Although a causal role can only be documented in prospective intervention trials, good indirect arguments have been advanced to indicate that the effect of blood pressure elevation on graft survival is a causal one. Although some studies failed to demonstrate that commonly recognized risk factors, particularly hypertension, are independently associated with the development of coronary artery disease in the post-transplant period [10], we suspect that the true impact of hypertension on cardiac survival was confounded by other factors in this study. If sensitive measurements, i.e. ambulatory BP measurement, are used, achieved blood pressure (with or without antihypertensive treatment) is high [17] in a large proportion of renal graft recipients followed for more than 6 months. Ambulatory BP values were strongly correlated, amongst others, to the rate of urinary albumin excretion in our study; confirming previous results of Lipkin [18] we noted a striking relation between mean ambulatory blood pressure and LVH. Some further information on blood pressure control is provided in Table 2. The difficulty of achieving blood pressure control is illustrated by the fact that in this patient population, the median number of antihypertensive agents used was no less than 3 (range 1–7).

Following a preliminary report by Horina and colleagues [19], regression of LVH during treatment with ACE inhibitors compared with placebo was confirmed by Lacalzada [20]. In 38 non-diabetic transplant recipients LVM decreased from a baseline value of 188 ± 11 to 173 ± 11 g/m². In the genesis of LVH and even cardiac death in uremic patients [21] increased aortic impedance as a result of reduced aortic elasticity plays an important role along with increased total peripheral resistance. In this context it is of interest that arterial distensibility remains significantly impaired in renal transplant recipients and this abnormality is related to the level of parathyroid hormone [22]. The impact of aortic elasticity on LV function is illustrated by the finding that a correlation exists between aortic elasticity and LVH in graft recipients. We and others found also a significant correlation between urinary albumin excretion and LVH, even in the range of microalbuminuria.

Table 2.   Achieved clinic blood pressure (median and range) in 90 long-term
(> 2 years) renal graft recipients in the outpatient clinic Heidelberg

Age (years)	48 (18–67)
Male/female	61/29
S-creatinine (mg/dl)	1.47 (0.83–8.1)
Systolic BP (mm/dl)	135 (110–180)
Diastolic BP (mm/Hg)	80 (60–105)
Patients on antihypertensive agents	81/90
Number of antihypertensive classes	3 (1–7)

No significant differences between genders,
Correlation between S-creatinine concentration and systolic ($r = 0.23$;
$p < 0.05$) or diastolic ($r = 0.22$; $p < 0.05$) blood pressure.
Antihypertensive agents: calcium channel blockers 77% of patients, diuretics
62%, betablockers 42%, ACE inhibitors or AT-II receptor antagonists 13%.

Dyslipoproteinemia

The presence of dyslipoproteinemia has been known since the early days of renal transplantation. A thorough review was provided by the late A. Raine [23]. Carotid plaques are frequent in renal transplant recipients [24] and in one study their frequency was even higher in transplanted patients with a history of cardiovascular events. Total cholesterol and diabetes mellitus were the only predictors of such cardiovascular events. In an analysis by Kasiske [12] ischemic heart disease was present in 20% of graft recipients after 15 years. Apart from age, presence of diabetes, male gender and episodes of rejection, lipids were independent predictors. The importance of lipids is illustrated by one impressive anecdotal observation [25] documenting that severe three vessel coronary heart disease in a graft recipient decreased during 2 years of LDL immunoadsorption treatment. The common presence of insulin resistance [26] may be an important contributor and also represent the common denominator in the genesis of post-transplant dyslipidemia and diabetes mellitus. Lp(a) is an independent predictor of cardiac death in hemodialyzed patients [27]. After transplantation a decrease of Lp(a) concentrations was reported by several authors [28], but whether after transplantation Lp(a) is also an independent predictor of cardiac risk has not been clarified.

Based on a priori considerations, Wanner et al. [29] advocated treatment with antilipidemic drugs in chronic allograft failure. There are good arguments that lipid lowering will reduce not only cardiac events [30], but also chronic allograft failure. This point is currently addressed in the ALERT study in the UK (assessment of Lescol in renal transplantation). The results will presumably also indicate whether cardiac risk is improved by statine treatment in this specific group of patients.

It has recently been shown that atherosclerosis is a microinflammatory state. It is conceivable that subthreshold inflammation in the graft promotes atherosclerosis in lesioned coronaries. This may explain the finding of Kasiske that rejection episodes have a significant impact on ischemic heart disease in graft recipients [12], although the alternative explanation that higher cumulative doses of steroids are responsible cannot be excluded.

Smoking

There is relatively little information on the impact of smoking on cardiovascular death in chronic graft recipients. Apart from some older reports, more recently Cosio [6] noted that smoking was a significant ($p < 0.009$) independent predictor of patient death in a cohort of 523 graft recipients with long-term (> 6 months) graft function.

Homocysteine

Hyperhomocysteinemia has been identified as a significant risk factor for cardiovascular disease in transplant recipients [31]. Plasma homocysteine concentrations were significantly higher than those in matched control subjects (15.5 ± 6.3 versus 8.7 ± 1.9 μmol/l, p 0.001). Patients with a history of vascular events had homocysteine concentrations >14 μmol/l more frequently (61%) than patients without (29%). Elevated homocysteine levels were confirmed by others who also noted a relationship with cyclosporin treatment [32], but the latter point is somewhat controversial [33]. It is conceivable that a potential effect of cyclosporin A is mediated via subtle changes of GFR. Since even a moderate elevation of homocysteine concentration, as noted in transplanted patients, is an independent risk factor for cardiovascular disease, it is of interest that a significant inverse relationship was noted between plasma homocysteine and plasma folate concentration. This observation suggests that folate supplementation may be a novel cardiac risk factor intervention in the future.

Interventions

Since pretransplant ischemic heart disease is a strong independent predictor of post-transplant cardiovascular events [12], it is certainly necessary to investigate prospective graft recipients according to the guidelines drawn up by the American Society of Transplant Physicians [34]. The appropriate procedures have been recently discussed in some detail [13].

There is currently no definite evidence from controlled prospective trials which document that therapeutic intervention reduce the rate of cardiovascular death in transplant recipients. Based on the above very strong circumstantial evidence it is certainly justified, however, to recommend a number of interventions, because their effectiveness is highly probable. To quote Sir William Osler 'clinical medicine is a science of uncertainty and an art of probability'.

We would suggest that blood pressure should be lowered at least to the levels recommended by JNC VI [14] for individuals with target organ damage, i.e. 130/85 mmHg. Blood pressure has a striking impact on late graft outcome [16], presumably analogous to that seen in primary glomerular disease [35]. Vasculitic graft injury may render the graft more susceptible to the effects of raised blood pressure. Based on these considerations we recommend even lower targets, i.e. 125/75 mmHg, as recently advocated by the National Kidney Foundation for patients with glomerular disease [36].

As to treatment of dyslipidemia, we offer the following thoughts. In diabetes mellitus the cardiac risk is increased by a factor of 3, and it has recently been argued [37] that statines are indicated in all diabetic patients, irrespective of the presence or absence of renal vascular disease, in view of the fact that baseline cardiac risk is so high. The situation is similar for patients with renal transplantation. According to B.C. Wheeler (personal communication) recipients of renal grafts in the UK have an annual cardiac death event rate of 2% compared to 3–4% for survivors of myocardial infarction. Since according to the Care Study [38], the effect of statines on reduction of cardiac events is independent of baseline serum cholesterol, it appears defensible to give statines either on a routine basis to all, or at least electively to all transplanted patients with a high cardiac risk profile, even in the absence of a clinical history of ischemic heart disease or overt hypercholesterolemia.

It is certainly wise to advise patients to stop smoking, although the efficacy of this advise must be viewed with some scepticism, given the fact that 20% of cardiac graft recipients continue to smoke according to our experience.

Since administration of moderate (5 mg/day) doses of folate does not cause toxicity, granted that vitamin B12 deficiency is excluded [39], it appears sensible to administer folate to graft recipients, at least if plasma homocysteine concentrations are above approximately 15 μmol/l. These interventions, designed to reduce the risk of cardiac disease, are also likely to protect the graft against progressive vascular injury. It is hoped that by these interventions one kills two birds with one stone, i.e. coronary disease and vascular disease of the graft.

References

1. Lindholm A, Albrechtsen D, Frödin L, Tufveson G, Persson NH, Lundgren G. Ischemic heart disease – major cause of death and graft loss after renal transplantation in Scandinavia. Transplantation. 1995; 60: 451–457.
2. Report on management of renal failure in Europe XXII, 1991. Nephrol. Dial. Transplant. 1992; 7(Suppl): 26.
3. Controlling the Epidemic of Cardiovascular Disease in Chronic Renal Disease: What Do We Know? What Do We Need to Learn? Where Do We Go from Here? Report from the National Kidney Foundation Task Force on Cardiovascular Disease. July 15, 1998.
4. Ojo AO, Port FK, Wolfe RA, Mauger EA, Williams L, Berling DP. Comparative mortality risks of chronic dialysis and cadaveric transplantation in black end-stage renal disease patients. Am. J. Kidney. Dis. 1994; 24: 59–64.

5. Bonal J, Clèries M, Vela E and the Renal Registry Committee. Transplantation versus haemodialysis in elderly patients. Nephrol. Dial. Transplant. 1997; 12: 261–264.
6. Cosio FG, Alamir A, Yim S et al. Patient survival after renal transplantation: 1. The impact of dialysis pre-transplant. Kidney Int. 1998; 53: 767–772.
7. Arend SM, Mallat MJ, Westendorp RJ, van der Woude FJ, van Es LA. Patient survival after renal transplantation; more than 25 years follow-up. Nephrol. Dial. Transplant. 1997; 12: 1672–1679.
8. McGregor E, Jardine AG, Murray LS et al. Pre-operative echocardiographic abnormalities and adverse outcome following renal transplantation. Nephrol. Dial. Transplant. 1998; 13: 1499–1505.
9. Surdacki A, Wieczorek Surdacka E, Sulowicz W, Dubiel JS. Effect of having a functioning cadaveric renal transplant on cardiovascular mortality risk in patients on renal replacement therapy. Nephrol. Dial. Transplant. 1995; 10: 1218–1223.
10. Hernandez D, Lacalzada J, Rufino M et al. Prediction of left ventricular mass changes after renal transplantation by polymorphism of the angiotensin-converting-enzyme gene. Kidney Int. 1997; 51: 1205–1211.
11. Parfrey PS, Harnett JD, Foley RN, Kent GM, Murray DC, Barre PE, Guttmann RD. Impact of renal transplantation on uremic cardiomyopathy. Transplantation. 1995; 60: 908–914.
12. Kasiske BL, Guijarro C, Massy ZA, Wiederkehr MR, Ma JZ. Cardiovascular disease after renal transplantation. J. Am. Soc. Nephrol. 1996; 7: 158–165.
13. Wheeler DC. Ischaemic heart disease after renal transplantation: how to assess and manage the risk. Nephrol. Dial. Transplant. (in press).
14. The Sixth Report of the Joint National Committee on Prevention, Detection, Evaluation, and Treatment of High Blood Pressure. National Institutes of Health, NIH Publication, No. 98-4080, November 1997.
15. Zeier M, Mandelbaum A, Ritz E. Hypertension in the transplanted patient. In: Contrib. Nephrol. 1998; 124: Basel: Karger: 1998.
16. Opelz G, Wujciak T, Ritz E. Association of chronic kidney graft failure with recipient blood pressure. Collaborative Transplant Study. Kidney Int. 1998; 53: 217–222.
17. Ambulante 24-Stunden-Blutdruckmessung (ABDM). Sektion Blutdruckmessung und Hochdruckdiagnostik der Deutschen Liga zur Bekämpfung des hohen Blutdruckes e.V., Deutsche Hypertonie Gesellschaft. Dtsch. Med. Wschr. 1998; 123: 1426–1430.
18. Lipkin GW, Tucker B, Giles M, Raine AE. Ambulatory blood pressure and left ventricular mass in cyclosporin- and non-cyclosporin-treated renal transplant recipients. J. Hypertens. 1993; 11: 439–442.
19. Horina JH, Zweiker R, Mauric A, Holzer H, Eber B. Regression of left ventricular hypertrophy (LVH) following renal transplantation. J. Am. Soc. Nephrol. 1994; 5: 1112.
20. Hernandez J, Lacalzada J, Linares J et al. Regression of left ventricular hypertrophy (LVH) by an angiotensin-converting-enzyme inhibitor (ACEI) after renal transplantation (RT). J. Am. Soc. Nephrol. 1997; 8: 714.
21. London GM. The concept of ventricular/vascular coupling: functional and structural alterations of the heart and arterial vessels go in parallel. Nephrol. Dial. Transplant. 1988; 13: 250–253.
22. Barenbrock M, Hausberg M, Kosch M, Kisters K, Hoeks APG, Rahn KH. Effect of hyperparathyroidism on arterial distensibility in renal transplant recipients. Kidney Int. 1998; 54: 210–215.
23. Raine AEG. Cardiovascular complications after renal transplantation. In Morris PJ, editor. Kidney Transplantation. Principles and Practice, 3rd edn. Philadelphia: W.B. Saunders Co.
24. Massy ZA, Mamzer-Bruneel MF, Chevalier A et al. Carotid atherosclerosis in renal transplant recipients. Nephrol. Dial. Transplant. 1998; 13: 1792–1798.
25. Jansen M, Gabriel H, Banyai S, Pidlich J, Weidinger F, Hörl WH, Derfler K. Regression of coronary atherosclerosis and amelioration of renal function during LDL-immunoadsorption therapy in a renal transplant recipient. Wien Klin. Wochenschr. 1996; 108: 425–431.
26. Midtvedt K, Hartmann A, Hjelmesaeth J, Lund K, Bjerkely BL. Insulin resistance is a common denominator of post-transplant diabetes mellitus and impaired glucose tolerance in renal-transplant recipients. Nephrol. Dial. Transplant. 1998; 13: 427–431.

27. Cressman MD, Heyka RJ, Paganini EP, O'Neil J, Skibinski CI, Hoff HF. Lipoprotein(a) is an independent risk factor for cardiovascular disease in hemodialysis patients. Circulation. 1992; 86: 475–482.
28. Webb AT, Reaveley DA, O'Donnell M, O'Connor B, Seed M, Brown EA. Lipids and lipo-protein(a) as risk factors for vascular disease in patients on renal replacement therapy. Nephrol. Dial. Transplant. 1995; 10: 354–357.
29. Wanner C, Bartens W, Galle J. Clinical utility of antiloipidemic therapies in chronic renal allograft failure. Kidney Int. 1995; 48(Suppl. 52): 60–62.
30. Kobashigawa JA, Katznelson S, Laks H et al. Effect of pravastatin on outcomes after cardiac transplantation. N. Engl. J. Med. 1995; 333: 621–627.
31. Massy ZA, Chadefaux-Vekemans B, Chevalier A et al. Hyperhomocysteinemia: a significant risk factor for cardiovaskular disease in renal transplant recipients. Nephrol. Dial. Transplant. 1994; 9: 1103–1108.
32. Arnadottir M, Hultberg B, Vladov V, Nilsson–Ehle P, Thysell H. Hyperhomocysteinemia in cyclosporin-treated renal transplant recipients. Transplantation. 1996; 61: 509–512.
33. Ducloux D, Ruedin C, Gibey R, Vautrin P, Bresson-Vautrin C, Rebibou JM, Chaloin JM. Prevalence determinants, and clinical significance of hyperhomocyst(e)inaemia in renal-transplant recipients. Nephrol. Dial. Transplant. 1998; 13: 2890–2893.
34. Kasiske BL, Ramos EL, Gaston RS. The evaluation of renal transplant candidates. Clinical practice guidelines. J. Am. Soc. Nephrol. 1995; 6: 1–34.
35. Peterson JC, Adler S, Burkart JM et al. Blood pressure control, proteinuria, and the progression of renal disease. The modification of diet in renal disease study. Ann. Intern. Med. 1995; 123: 754–762.
36. Jacobson HR, Striker GE. Report on a workshop to develop management recommendations for the prevention of progression in chronic renal disease. Am. J. Kidney Dis. 1995; 25: 103–106.
37. Haffner SM, Letho S, Rönnemaa TM, Pyörälä K, Laakso M. Mortality from coronary heart disease in subjects with type 2 diabetes and in nondiabetic subjects with and without prior myocardial infarction. N. Engl. J. Med. 1998; 339: 229–234.
38. Sacks FM, Pfeffer MA, Moye LA et al. The effect of pravastatin on coronary events after myocardial infarction in patients with average cholesterol levels. Cholesterol and recurrent events trial investigators. N. Engl. J. Med. 1996; 335: 1001–1009.
39. Westhuyzen J. Folate supplementation in the dialysis patient – fragmentary evidence and tentative recommendations. Nephrol. Dial. Transplant. 1998; 13: 2748–2750.

11. Strategies to minimize nephrotoxicity associated to calcineurin inhibitors

J. ALSINA

Introduction

During the last decades the increasing importance of the dose-related acute and chronic nephrotoxic effects of calcineurin inhibitors (CNI), namely cyclosporine and tacrolimus has been reported [1–3]. Mihatsch et al. [4] found that the side effect pattern of these drugs is nearly identical: they were unable to differentiate morphological changes associated with their clinical nephrotoxicity.

It is also important to consider that broad experimental and clinical evidence demonstrate that nephron mass supply as well as recipient metabolic demand are both important predictors of graft survival [5, 6]. Moreover, taking into account that ischemia–reperfusion injury plays also an important role in the cadaveric allograft setting, donor nephron mass becomes susceptible for additional important losses. The magnitude of this initial damage may further increase whenever acute rejection or early post-transplantation acute nephrotoxicity episodes occur.

Acute nephrotoxicity of calcineurin inhibitors

Acute CNI nephrotoxicity induces renal vasoconstriction which leads to a reduction of renal plasma flow, glomerular filtration rate and natriuresis. Several factors previously reported to mediate CNI-induced vasoconstriction, include adrenergic mediators and the renin-angiotensin axis [7–9]. Recently, Amore et al. [10] showed that initial vasoconstriction depends upon an imbalance between the various modulators of the renal vascular tone, among which endothelins and nitric oxide seem to be the most powerful. However, these functional abnormalities are reversible post-transplantation whenever CNI are withdrawn [11]. Another important consequence of vasoconstriction is that it contributes to the high frequency of hypertension observed in these patients, and endothelin (ET) may play a pivotal role [12].

It was previously thought that the reversibility of CNI vasoconstriction was limited to the early stages of renal transplantation. Interestingly, Ader et al. [13] have recently shown that renal allografts are capable of retaining a good functional reserve in surviving stable CsA-treated kidney transplant recipients

P. Cochat et al. (eds.), Immunosuppression under Trial, 89–99
©1999 Kluwer Academic Publishers.

beyond the first year after grafting. Thus, these authors have shown that the renal functional reserve represents 21% and 22% of the baseline glomerular filtration rate 2 and 4 years post-transplantation. They suggest that renal vasoconstriction is still partially reversible at these stages and indicate that the graft does not exhibit a permanent glomerular hyerfiltration.

Recent body of evidence demonstrates that CsA induces TGF-β1 expression [14] and that TGF-β1 stimulates endothelin production [15]. Interestingly, Dogu et al. [16] showed that prostaglandin E1 inhibits CsA-induced up-regulation of TGF-β1. Moreover, other strategies can also down-regulate TGF-β1 expression. Thus, Islam et al. [17] neutralized TGF-β1 effect by employing an anti-TGF-β1 antibody. They prevented both a creatinine clearance fall and CsA-mediated arteriolar hyalinosis in an experimental model, and they concluded that certain nephrotoxic features were clearly mediated by TGF-β1.

Strategies to minimize acute CNI nephrotoxicity

In order to properly decrease the long-term effects of acute CNI nephrotoxicity, we have to bear in mind that different inter-related factors may have additive deleterious effects on kidney allograft survival [18]. Thus, the confluence of different risk factors such as elder donors or prolonged cold ischemia times will definitely influence preventive therapeutic approaches.

Among several possibilities, the first potential approach would be the use of different drugs with a beneficial effect on ischemia–reperfusion damage [19]. The most promising to date are shown in Table 1 [19–32].

Since the different pathophysiological mechanisms triggered during ischemia–reperfusion are likely to contribute to the development of chronic transplant nephropathy (CTN), any attempt to diminish early allograft injury may certainly improve long-term graft outcome.

Table 1.   Drug approach to minimize CNI-induced nephrotoxicity and ischemia–reperfusion damage

PAF antagonists	[19]
Oxigen free-radical scavengers: i.e. superoxidismutase	[20]
Monoclonal antibodies: i.e. anti LFA-1	[21]
Antisense oligodeoxynucleotides: i.e. anti ICAM-1	[22, 23]
Endothelin receptor antagonists	[24, 25]
Nitric oxide donors	[26, 27]
Eicosapentanoic acid	[28]
21-aminosteroid U 74389 G	[29]
Glycine	[30]
Angiotensin-converting enzyme inhibitors	[31]
Angiotensin II receptor antagonists	[31]
Prostacyclin	[32]

Long-term consequences of early CNI nephrotoxicity

This issue remains highly controversial but it may well be of paramount importance. Solez et al. [33] described a higher occurrence of CTN among those patients who experienced previous episodes of clinical CsA nephrotoxicity when they analyzed 144 protocol biopsies performed 2 years after transplantation. We also have data supporting a potential long-term damaging effect of early CsA exposure [34, 35]. Thus, in 282 clinically stable patients (creatinine < 300 mmol/l and proteinuria <1 g/l) who underwent a 3-month protocol biopsy, early CsA exposure until biopsy was independently associated with the presence of CTN according to the Banff criteria. Moreover, when a logistic regression analysis was performed, donor age, cold ischemia time and acute rejection were also independent predictors of CTN together with CsA exposure. Interestingly, mean CsA levels were within the normal therapeutic range (231 ± 74 ng/ml in the CTN group versus 206 ± 73 in the normal group). Therefore, it is possible that even seemingly normal levels of CsA might have deleterious effects on graft fibrosis and the use of the lowest CsA dose compatible with efficient immunosuppression should be recommended. The presence or absence of early damage in these protocol biopsies also predicts long-term allograft outcome. Thus, in the group of 174 patients with normal histology, 10-year graft survival was as high as 95.4%. On the other hand, in the group of 87 patients which had shown CTN, in the absence of transplant-associated vasculopathy (TAV), 10-year graft survival was 82.3%, whereas in the 21 patients with CTN and TAV (chronic rejection) graft survival was much lower (41.3%; p < 0.0001) [35].

Immunosuppressive strategies to minimize early CNI exposure

Some groups initially tried to assess the efficacy of CNI-free induction protocols when managing patients receiving suboptimal grafts, where it would not be wise to expose them to a potential additional damaging factor. Therefore, a new array of non-nephrotoxic immunosuppressive agents have been introduced in clinical practice, including mycophenolate mofetil (MMF) and anti IL-2R monoclonal antibodies. The availability of these new drugs has further allowed the use of these protocols in patients with delayed graft function or those who show at a later time clinical or histological evidence of CNI nephrotoxicity.

It is well known that allografts from suboptimal donors are associated with a higher incidence of delayed graft function [36, 37] and that these grafts are more susceptible to CNI nephrotoxicity [38]. We have recently reported our experience on 17 non-sensitized recipients of a suboptimal graft [39]. The immunosuppressive induction protocol was based on five alternate doses of antithymocyte globulin plus MMF and steroids avoiding the use of CNI. As a maintenance treatment, patients were treated with MMF and steroids. Delayed graft function occurred in 12% of cases. Biopsy-proven acute rejection episodes were diagnosed in 24%. Cyclosporine was added in three out of these four cases with acute rejection. All patients were alive with a functioning allograft after 6 months of follow-up. Mean serum creatinine was 159 ± 59 mmol/l. In this study, we have shown that this protocol is efficient and can avoid the use of CsA in 70% of patients.

Before the appearance of these new non-nephrotoxic drugs, two strategies were employed to decrease the nephrotoxic effects of CNI during the early post-transplant period: the delayed introduction of CsA in the so-called sequential induction protocols [40–42]; or the use of concomitant low doses of CsA [43–45]. Both induction regimens are associated with the use of antilymphocytic polyclonal or monoclonal antibodies. Long-term renal allograft outcome in patients treated with prophylactic antilymphocyte globulin or OKT3 is significantly superior when compared with standard triple therapy [46,47]. With the advent of new immunosupresants (MMF, rapamycin and monoclonal antibodies against IL-2R) novel sequential or concomitant protocols may be designed using even lower doses of CNI.

Chronic nephrotoxicity of calcineurin inhibitors

There is a quite general agreement that the main risk factors related to chronic graft dysfunction are donor-related risk factors, such as age > 50 years and/or the presence of a reduced nephron mass; ischemia–reperfusion injury secondary to prolonged cold ischemia times; severe acute rejection-mediated renal damage; and acute and/or chronic CNI-induced nephrotoxicity. The main target of these damaging pathways leading to chronic graft dysfunction is the renal vasculature. Myers et al. [48] reported 10 years ago the appearance of CsA-induced nephrotoxicity in a group of 37 cardiac transplant patients treated with high CsA doses for 12–24 months. They found increased renal vascular resistance, decreased glomerular filtration rate, proteinuria and hypertension. Common pathological findings were obliterative arteriolopathy and tubulointerstitial damage. This chronic CsA damage was rarely reversible and potentially progressive.

Which are the mechanisms leading to CNI-induced chronic nephrotoxicity? We know that CNI cause a dose-related decrease in renal function secondary to afferent arteriolar vasoconstriction. It is believed that the chronic persistence of this state of renal vasoconstriction leading to tissue ischemia might be responsible for the development of chronic CNI toxicity. Pascual et al. [49] have stated that chronic rejection and chronic CsA toxicity share a common pathophysiological pathway leading to progressive allograft failure. They speculate that prolonged and sustained expression of TGF-β1 after the first 6 months post-transplantation might participate in the pathogenesis of CTN.

Nevertheless, we have to bear in mind that CNI exert also beneficial and essential immunosupressive effects, such as down-regulation of T-cell promoting genes (i.e. IL-2) as well as an increase in the production of TGF-β1 [50].

Both pathways contribute to the immunosuppressive effect of CNI. However, as mentioned above, the increase in TGF-$\beta1$ could contribute both to renal scarring and ET-1-mediated hypertension, which in turn may aggravate the direct stimulatory effect of CsA on sympathetic activity. It is not yet known whether different CNI have distinct effects on TGF-$\beta1$ synthesis.

Strategies to minimize chronic nephrotoxicity induced by anticalcineurin agents

Maintenance protocols without anticalcineurin agents

Beyond the previously mentioned protocols used for suboptimal donors, some groups have employed new non-nephrotoxic immunosuppressants without CNI in conventional primary cadaveric kidney transplantation. Similarly to anticalcineurin agents, a recently developed humanized anti IL-2R monoclonal antibody (Daclizumab, DZB) also interferes with IL-2 synthesis. Its homology to humans explains the very prolonged therapeutic effect of this drug. On behalf of the DZB/MMF Combination Renal Transplant Study [51], Grinyó reported promising results with the combination of DZB, MMF and steroids, without CNI, in recipients of first renal allografts. Five doses of DZB were given intravenously every 2 weeks and MMF was initially given orally at 3 g/day and tapered to 2 g/day after 6 months. Acute rejection episodes appeared in 27% of patients who then received CNI. This protocol seems to be an effective and safe non-nephrotoxic immunosuppressive regimen that may avoid the use of CNI in almost 75% of treated patients.

Calcineurin inhibitor conversion to mycophenolate mofetil

A different approach is represented by those protocols which use CNI during the early phase post-transplantation, but then switch a to a non-nephrotoxic drug [52, 53]. It is noteworthy that the later CNI is switched to MMF, the lower the likelihood of late acute rejection episodes. Houde et al. [54] reported 10 patients with biopsy-proven CsA nephrotoxicity who were switched from CsA to MMF 4 years after transplantation. In this study, all patients increased their creatinine clearance whereas no episodes of acute rejection were observed. On the other hand, Schrama et al. [52] and Van Gelder et al. [53] performed an earlier switch, 6 or 12 months post-transplantation, respectively. In both studies, the conversion of CsA to MMF was safe in the vast majority of patients and was followed by an improvement of renal hemodynamics, blood pressure and serum uric acid. Unfortunately, some patients experienced acute rejection episodes but these were either steroid-sensitive or responsive to the reintroduction of CsA. Long-term functional effects of these early conversions remain a matter of discussion.

Maintenance therapies with low doses of calcineurin inhibitors   In an attempt to minimize chronic CNI nephrotoxicity and analyze its potential reversibility, several authors significantly reduced the previous administered CsA doses in patients with suspected chronic CNI nephrotoxicity. Thus, Mourad et al. [55] assessed 23 renal transplant patients with biopsy-proven CsA nephropathy who were followed for more than 2 years either after a CsA dose reduction (18 patients) or CsA withdrawal (five patients) associated with the introduction of azathioprine. They observed a significant increase in the glomerular filtration rate and renal plasma flow, as well as a significant decrease in serum creatinine. Only one episode of acute reversible rejection was recorded. Nevertheless, chronic rejection developed in three cases.

Other groups have recently reported the use of MMF in this context [56, 57]. We have evaluated the impact of CsA reduction associated with MMF introduction, both on TGF-β1 production and renal function in 18 long-term stable renal allograft recipients with suspected CsA nephrotoxicity. The CsA dose was reduced to reach whole-blood levels between 40 and 60 ng/mL within one month. The introduction of MMF allowed us to decrease significantly the CsA dose and CsA levels, and an increase in both the glomerular filtration rate and renal plasma flow was recorded. We also showed for the first time in humans that this manoeuver was followed by a reduction in plasma TGF-β1 levels (from 4.6 to 2 ng/ml; $p = -0.003$). Cyclosporine levels were positively correlated with TGF-β1 levels (R = 0.536, $p = 0.002$). We observed no rejection episodes and there was a significant improvement in both systolic and diastolic blood pressure [56]. Weir et al. [57] followed a similar approach in a group of patients with histologically proven CTN. They added MMF, halved the dose of CsA and observed an improvement of renal function in 21 out of 28 patients in the absence of acute rejection episodes. Thus, we believe that a CNI dose reduction should not be limited to the patients with a clear-cut biopsy-proven CNI nephrotoxicity or CTN, but it could be also attempted in patients with a progressive deterioration of renal function (namely chronic graft dysfunction), provided that no signs of ongoing acute rejection are present. Nevertheless, in cases with stable suboptimal renal function (i.e. serum creatinine between 140 and 300 mmol/l, proteinuria 1 g/day) we think that a biopsy is not mandatory.

Hong Song et al. [58] have confirmed by immunohistochemical staining of renal allograft biopsies that chronic reduction of CsA may diminish the production of TGF-β1 and they have also shown that this manoeuver decreases the expression of TGF-β1 receptor. It results in a decreased collagen synthesis and stabilization or improvement of fibrosis in the tissue of patients with CTN.

Interference with molecular signals leading to scarring

Antagonizing TGF-β1 production: Since direct antagonism of TGF-β1 effects is not yet clinically available, an indirect strategy has been recently reported. Peters et al. [59] demonstrated that both an angiotensin I converting enzyme inhibitor (enalapril) and the angiotensin II receptor blocker losartan reduced TGF-β1 overproduction in an experimental rat model of glomerulonephritis. Furthermore, Campistol et al. [60] have shown that treatment of hypertensive renal transplant patients with losartan not only achieved control of hypertension and a fall in urinary protein excretion but also significantly decreased the levels of TGF-β1 and ET-1. We do not know yet whether these drugs will help to limit CNI nephrotoxicity by interfering these pathways.

Modulating extracellular matrix metabolism and decreasing interstitial cellular activity: Investigation of the molecular events that lead to renal fibrosis in rodent models indicate that different pathways may be at work, such as up-regulation of TGF-β1 and disturbances in extracellular matrix turnover, as well as infiltration of cells of the macrophage/monocyte lineage. Duymelinck et al. [61] reported an increased expression of tissue inhibitor of matrix metallo-proteinase type 1 (TIMP1) in the kidneys of CsA-treated rats, in parallel with a marked influx of macrophages/monocytes in the damaged renal areas.

The results of this study suggested that the intrarenal inhibition of matrix degradation in the kidney, rather than a decrease of protease expression, would contribute to CNI nephrotoxicity. Moreover, the recruitment of macrophages, linked to CsA dose, appeared to be critical in the progression of CsA-induced interstitial fibrosis.

On the other hand, it seems that MMF may attenuate macrophage infiltration in a remnant kidney rat model, and this drug largely diminished glomerular and interstitial injury [62]. Hence, in addition to its immunosuppressive properties, MMF may have beneficial non-immunological effects that might further attenuate CNI toxicity.

Minimizing transplant vasculopathy: We have previously discussed the potential strategies to decrease vascular injury related to ischemia–reperfusion damage and we have also underlined the importance of an efficient and non-nephrotoxic immunosuppression. However, the important relationship between lipids and transplant vasculopathy remains to be characterized. Many groups have reported the presence of an association between the pre- or post-transplant cholesterol levels and chronic rejection [63–65]. Importantly, our group has shown that total serum cholesterol before transplantation was the only independent predictor for the development of early transplant vasculopathy [35]. Thus, lipid-mediated damage might also contribute to the appearance and/or progression of chronic rejection. Total serum cholesterol could, therefore, be another potential target to modify the natural history of transplant vasculopathy. In this regard, in addition to the previous recommendations to minimize ischemia–reperfusion injury, expression of potentially deleterious chemical mediators or cellular events, it is possible that renal transplant patients could also benefit of an early treatment with statins [35]. Moreover, it has been shown recently that statins may inhibit progressive chronic vascular rejection in rat cardiac allografts, and that they may act by mechanisms other than their effects on the lipid profile [66]. Thus, statins may also modulate extracellular matrix turnover and block macrophage infiltration.

References

1. Myers BD. Cyclosporine nephrotoxicity. Kidney Int. 1986; 30: 964–974.
2. Cole E, Keown P, Landsberg D et al. Safety and tolerability of cyclosporine and cyclosporine microemulsion during 18 months of follow-up in stable renal transplant recipients: a report of the Canadian Neoral Renal Study Group. Transplantation. 1998; 65: 505–510.
3. Katari SR, Magnone M, Shapiro R et al. Clinical features of acute reversible tacrolimus (FK 506) nephrotoxicity in kidney transplant recipients. Clin. Transplant. 1997; 11: 237–242.
4. Mihatsch MJ, Kyo M, Morozumi K, Yamagushi Y, Nickeleit V, Ryfeel B. The side-effects of ciclosporine-A and tacrolimus. Clin. Nephrol. 1998; 49: 356–363.
5. Azuma H, Nadeau K, Mackenzie HS, Brenner BM, Tilney NL. Nephron mass modulates the hemodynamic, cellular, and molecular response of the rat renal allograft. Transplantation. 1997; 63: 519–528.
6. Moreso F, Serón D, Anunciada AI et al. Recipient body surface area as a predictor of post–transplant renal allograft evolution. Transplantation. 1998; 65: 671–676.
7. Moss NG, Powell SI, Falk RJ. Intravenous cyclosporin activates afferent and efferent nerves and causes sodium retention in innervated kidney in rats. Proc. Natl. Acad. Sci. USA. 1985; 82: 8226–8226.
8. Kaskel FS, Deverajan P, Arbeit La, Partin JS, Moore LC. Cyclosporin nephrotoxicity: Sodium excretion, autoregulation and angiotensin II. Am. J. Physiol. 1987; 252: F733–F742.
9. Perico N, Benigni A, Bosco E, Remuzzi G. Acute cyclosporin A nephrotoxicity in rats: which role for renin-angiotensin system and glomerular prostaglandins? Clin. Nephrol. 1996; 25: S83–S88.
10. Amore A, Gianoglio B, Ghigo D et al. A possible role for nitric oxide in modulating the functional cyclosporine toxicity by arginine. Kidney Int. 1995; 47: 1507–1514.
11. Bennett WM, De Mattos A, Meyer MM, Andoh T, Barry JM. Chronic cyclosporine nephropathy: the Achilles' heel of immunosuppressive therapy. Kidney Int. 1996; 50: 1089–1100.
12. Meyer-Lehnert H, Bokemeyer D, Friedrichs U, Backer A, Kramer HJ. Cellular mechanisms of cyclosporine A-associated side-effects: role of endothelin. Kidney Int. Suppl. 1997; 61: S27–S31.
13. Ader JL, Rostaing L, Tran-van T, Tack Y, Cisterne JM, Durand D. Persistence of a renal functional reserve at four years after transplantation in surviving cyclosporine-treated kidney recipients. J. Am. Soc. Nephrol. 1998; 9: 661A.
14. Khanna A, Kapur S, Sharma V, Li B, Suthanthiran M. In vivo hyperexpression of transforming growth factor-β1 in mice: stimulation by cyclosporine. Transplantation. 1997; 63: 1037–1039.
15. Kirk AD, Jacobson LM, Heisey DM, Fass NA, Sollinger HW, Pirsch JD. Postransplant diastolic hypertension: associations with intragraft transforming growth factor β1, endothelin, and renin transcription. Transplantation. 1997; 64: 1716–1720.
16. Dogu E, Waiser J, Gaedeke J, Bohler T, Budde K, Neumayer HH. PGE1 prevents cyclosporine-induced upregulation of TGF-β1 in rat mesangial cells. J. Am. Soc. Nephrol. 1998; 9: 649A.
17. Islam M, Burke JF, Francos GC, Sharma K. Effect of anti-TGF-β1 antibody on kidneys of cyclosporine (CyA) treated rats. J. Am. Soc. Nephrol. 1998; 9: 652A.
18. Grinyo JM, Gil-Vernet S, Moreso F et al. Ischemia-reperfusion injury as a risk factor for late kidney graft failure. In: Touraine JL et al. (eds). Late Graft Loss. London: Kluwer Academic Publishers, 1997: 77–83.
19. Grinyo JM. BN 52021: a platelet activating factor antagonist for preventing post-transplant renal failure. A double-blind, randomized study. The BN 52021 Study Group in Renal Transplantation. Ann. Intern. Med. 1994; 121: 345–347.

20. Land W, Schneeberger H, Schleibner S et al. The beneficial effect of human recombinant superoxide dismutase on acute and chronic rejection events in recipients of cadaveric renal transplants. Transplantation. 1994; 57: 211–217.

21. Hourmant M, Bedrossian J, Durand D et al. A randomized multicenter trial comparing leukocyte function-associated antigen-1 monoclonal antibody with rabbit antithymocyte globulin as induction treatment in first kidney transplantations. Transplantation. 1996; 62: 1565–1570.

22. Haller H, Dragun D, Miethke A et al. Antisense oligonucleotides for ICAM-1 attenuate reperfusion injury and renal failure in the rat. Kidney Int. 1996; 50: 473–480.

23. Stepkowski SM, Wang M, Condon TP et al. Protection against allograft rejection with intercellular adhesion molecule-1 antisense oligodeoxynucleotides. Transplantation. 1998; 66: 699–707.

24. Gellai M, Jugus M, Fletcher T, DeWolf R, Nambi P. Reversal of postischemic acute renal failure with a selective endothelin-A receptor antagonist in the rat. J. Clin. Invest. 1994; 93: 900–906.

25. Herrero I, Torras J, Riera M et al. Prevention of cold ischemia-reperfusion injury by an endothelin receptor antagonist in experimental transplantation. Nephrol. Dial. Transplant. 1999; 14: 872–880.

26. Siegfried MR, Erhardt J, Rider T, Ma XL, Lefer AM. Cardioprotection and attenuation of endothelial dysfunction by organic nitric oxide donors in myocardial ischemia–reperfusion. J. Pharmacol. Exp. Ther. 1992; 260: 668–675.

27. Andoh TF, Gardner MP, Bennett WM. Protective effects of dietary l-arginine supplementation on chronic cyclosporine nephrotoxicity. Transplantation. 1997; 64: 1236–1240.

28. Torras J, Soto K, Riera M et al. Changes in renal hemodynamics and physiology after normothermic ischemia in animals supplemented with eicosapentaenoic acid. Transplant. Int. 1996; 9 (Suppl 1): S455–S459.

29. Shoskes DA, Jones E, Garras N, Satyanarayana K. Effect of the lazaroid U-74389G on chemokine gene expression and apoptosis in renal ischemia-reperfusion injury. Transplant. Proc. 1998; 30: 974–975.

30. Thurman RG, Zhong Z, von Frankenberg M, Stachlewitz RF, Bunzendahl H. Prevention of cyclosporine-induced nephrotoxicity with dietary glycine. Transplantation. 1997; 63: 1661–1667.

31. Amore A, Cirina P, Conti G, Peruzzi L, Ricotti E, Fiorucci GC. Coppo R. ACE inhibitors and Angiotensin II receptor antagonists (ATI-RA) inhibit apoptosis induced by cyclosporin A. J. Am. Soc. Nephrol. 1998; 9: 646A.

32. Hansen JM, Christensen NJ, Fogh-Andersen N, Strandgaard S. Effects of the prostacyclin analogue iloprost on cyclosporin-induced renal hypoperfusion in stable renal transplant recipients. Nephrol. Dial. Transplant. 1996; 11: 340–346.

33. Solez K, Vincenti F, Filo R and the US FK506 Kidney Transplant Study Group. Histopathologic findings from 2-year protocol biopsies from a U.S. Multicenter Kidney Transplant trial comparing Tacrolimus versus cyclosporine. Transplantation. 1998; 66: 1736–1740.

34. Serón D, Moreso F et al. Early protocol renal allograft biopsies and graft outcome. Kidney Int. 1997; 51: 310–316.

35. Seron D, Moreso F, Ramon JM et al. Protocol renal allograft biopsies in the design of clinical trials aimed to improve late graft outcome. Submitted.

36. Gaston RS, Schlessinger SD. Delayed graft function after transplantation: causes, implications, and clinical management. J. Nephrol. 1994; 7: 313–321.

37. Gaber LW, Moore LW, Alloway RR, Amiri MH, Vera SR, Gaber AO. Glomerulosclerosis as a determinant of posttransplant function of older donor renal allografts. Transplantation. 1995; 60: 334–339.

38. Leunissen KM, Bosman FT, Nieman FH, Kootstra G, Vromen MA, Noordzij TC, van Hooff JP. Amplification of the nephrotoxic effect of cyclosporine by preexistent chronic histological lesions in the kidney. Transplantation. 1989; 48: 590–593.

39. Grinyó JM, Gil-Vernet S, Serón D et al. Primary immunosuppression with mycophenolate mofetil and antithymocyte globulin for kidney transplant recipients of a suboptimal graft. Nephrol. Dial. Transplant. 1998; 13: 2601–2604.

40. Stratta RJ, D'Alessandro AM, Armbrust MJ, Pirsch JD, Sollinger HW, Kalayoglu M, Belzer FO. Sequential antilymphocyte globulin/cyclosporine immunosuppression in cadaveric renal transplantation. Effect of duration of ALG therapy. Transplantation. 1989; 47: 96–102.

41. Norman DJ, Kahana L, Stuart FP Jr et al. A randomized clinical trial of induction therapy with OKT3 in kidney transplantation. Transplantation. 1993; 55: 44–50.

42. Cole EH, Cattran DC, Farewell VT et al. A comparison of rabbit antithymocyte serum and OKT3 as prophylaxis against renal allograft rejection. Transplantation. 1994; 57: 60–67.

43. Griño JM, Alsina J, Sabater R et al. Antilymphoblast globulin, cyclosporine, and steroids in cadaveric renal transplantation. Transplantation. 1990; 49: 114–1117.

44. Griñó JM, Castelao AM, Serón D et al. Antilymphocyte globulin versus OKT3 induction therapy in cadaveric kidney transplantation: a prospective randomized study. Am. J. Kidney Dis. 1992; 20: 603–610.

45. Zietse R, van Steenberge EP, Hesse CJ, Vaessen LB, Ijzermans JN, Weimar W. Single-shot, high-dose rabbit ATG for rejection prophylaxis after kidney transplantation. Transplant. Int. 1993; 6: 337–340.

46. Alsina J, Bover J, Gil-Vernet S et al. Longterm allograft outcome in patients treated with prophylactic antilymphoctye globulin or OKT3 as induction therapy in cadaveric kidney transplantation. In: Touraine JL et al. (eds) Late Graft Loss. Dordrecht: Kluwer Academic Publishers; 1997: 111–120.

47. Shield CF, Edwards EB, Davies DB, Daily OP. Antilymphocyte induction therapy in cadaver renal transplantation: a retrospective, multicenter United Network for Organ Sharing Study. Transplantation. 1997; 63: 1257–1263.

48. Myers BD, Sibley R, Newton L et al. The long-term course of cyclosporine-associated chronic nephropathy. Kidney Int. 1988; 33: 590–600.

49. Pascual M, Swinford RD, Ingelfinger JR, Williams WW, Cosimi AB, Tolkoff-Rubin N. Chronic rejection and chronic cyclosporin toxicity in renal allografts. Immunol. Today. 1998; 19: 514–519.

50. Shin GT, Khanna A, Ding R, Sharma VK, Lagman M, Li B, Suthanthiran M. In vivo expression of transforming growth factor-betal in humans: stimulation by cyclosporine. Transplantation. 1998; 65: 313–318.

51. Vincenti F, Grinyó J, Ramos E et al. Can antibody prophylaxis allow sparing of other immunosuppressives? Transplant Proc. 1999; 31: 1246.

52. Schrama YC, Hené RJ, Boer P, Koomans HA. Conversion of cyclosporine (neoral) to mycophenolate mofetil (cellcept) in stable renal transplant patients. Transplantation. 1998; 65 (Suppl.) 184.

53. van Gelder T, de Kuiper P, van Besouw NM, van der Mast B, Gregoor PJHS, Ijzermans JNM, Weimar W. Randomised trial comparing conversion of maintenance treatment with cyclosporine and prednisone to azathioprine or mycophenolate mofetil with predisone one year after kidney transplantation. Transplantation. 1998; 65 (Suppl): 140.

54. Houde Y, Noel R, de Cotret PR, Boucher D, Lachance JG. Prednisone-mycophenolate mofetil double therapy for cyclosporine a toxicity in kidney transplantation. Transplantation. 1998; 65 (Suppl): 139.

55. Mourad G, Vela C, Ribstein J, Mimran A. Long-term improvement in renal function after cyclosporine reduction in renal transplant recipients with histologically proven chronic cyclosporine nephropathy. Transplantation. 1998; 65: 661–667.

56. Hueso M, Bover J, Serón et al. Low-dose cyclosporine and mycophenolate mofetil in renal allograft recipients with suboptimal renal function. Transplantation. 1998; 66: 1727–1731.

57. Weir MR, Anderson L, Fink JC et al. A novel approach to the treatment of chronic allograft nephropathy. Transplantation. 1997; 64: 1706–1710.

58. Hong Song, Seta K, Papadimitriou JC, Drachenberg CI, Weir MR, Wei CM. Chronic reduction of cyclosporine results in reduced expression of transforming growth factor-beta and its receptor isoforms in renal biopsies of patients with chronic allograft nephropathy. J. Am. Soc. Nephrol. 1998; 9: 657A.

59. Peters H, Border WA, Noble NA. Targeting TGF β1 overexpression in renal disease: Maximizing the antifibrotic action of angiotensin II blockade. Kidney Int. 1998; 54: 1570–1580.
60. Campistol JM, Inigo P, Lario S, Jimenez W, Clesca PH, Oppenheimer F, Rivera F. Angiotensin II receptor antagonist (Losartan) decreases plasma levels of TGF-β1 in transplant patients with chronic allograft nephropathy. Kidney Int. 1999 (in press)
61. Duymelinck C, Deng JT, Dauwe SEH, De Broe ME, Verpooten GA. Inhibition of the matrix metalloproteinase system in a rat model of chronic cyclosporine nephropathy. Kidney Int. 1998; 54: 804–818.
62. Fujihara CK, Costa Malheiros DM, Zatz R, Noronha L. Mycophenolate mofetil attenuates renal injury in the rat remnant kidney. Kidney Int. 1998; 54: 1510–1519.
63. Markell MS, Sumrani N, Dibenedetto A, Friedman EA. Effect of early hyperlipidemia on graft and patient survival in cyclosporine-treated renal transplant patients. Am. J. Kidney Dis. 1993; 22: 233–239.
64. Dimény E, Tufveson G, Lithell H, Larsson E, Siegbahn A, Fellstrom B. The influence of pretransplant lipoprotein abnormalities in the early results of renal transplantation. Eur. J. Clin. Invest. 1993; 23: 572–579.
65. Massy ZA, Guijarro C, Wiederkehr MR, Ma JZ, Kasiske BL. Chronic allograft rejection: Immunological and nonimmunological risk factors. Kidney Int. 1996; 49: 518–524.
66. Maggard MA, Ke B, Wang T, Kaldas F, Seu P, Busuttil RW, Imagawa DK. Effects of pravastatin on chronic rejection of rat cardiac allografts. Transplantation. 1998; 65: 149–155.

12. Diabetogenic effect of immunosuppressive drugs

X. MARTIN

Introduction

Many immunosuppressive drugs to show either experimental or clinical effects on glucose metabolism and regulation. These can arise from either a direct toxic effect on islet beta cells, or an indirect effect, such as insulin resistance. The problem of immunosuppression-induced diabetes is clinically relevant because patients may develop long-term degenerative complications related to glucose intolerance or suffer a deterioration of their quality of life resulting from a need for insulin injections and strict diet, an unexpected restriction in a transplanted patient with a functional organ. Disorders of glucose metabolism may also enhance complications induced by some other metabolic abnormalities found in transplant recipients, such as atherosclerosis and disorders in lipid metabolism. The diabetic state can decompensate or accelerate cardiovascular complications, which is a leading cause of patient death after transplantation.

Steroids have been widely used for immunosuppression and are very well known as inducers of insulin resistance, but other new very potent drugs are also responsible for a post-transplant diabetic state. New immunosuppressive regimens are designed to lower this diabetogenic effect. We will review the different options for reducing this detrimental effect.

Diabetogenic effect of different drugs

Steroids have been used since the very beginning of transplantation, and are still used for induction, maintenance and treatment of acute rejection. Disorders of glucose metabolism occur as a side effect of steroids. Steroids induce a post-receptor defect of the action of insulin, which is inseparable from the therapeutic effect. Patients on steroid therapy usually show a 2-fold increase in insulin secretion. In most cases no treatment is required, as glucose levels remain subnormal. In some categories of patients, such as the obese or elderly, hyperglycemia is observed after transplantation. Hyperglycemia may be important and associated with ketoacidosis, insulin therapy then has to be started. Decreasing steroid dosages to the usual 5–15 mg/day is usually associated with a decrease in insulin requirement and even a switch to oral hypoglycemic drugs.

P. Cochat et al. (eds.), Immunosuppression under Trial, 101–103
©1999 Kluwer Academic Publishers.

Calcineurin inhibitors

Cyclosporine A and FK 506 share the same molecular mechanism of action: inhibition of calcineurin phosphatase activity and of the calcineurin NF-AT signaling which is necessary for the transcription of the IL2 gene [1]. The mechanisms involved in β-cell toxicity are not well documented. Cyclosporine inhibits insulin secretion in rats and in human β-cells [2], but its toxicity is reversible. FK 506 had a frank diabetogenic effect in some clinical trials. Tolerance tests performed on liver transplanted patients after withdrawal of steroids showed that according to WHO criteria, 40% of liver transplant recipients have glucose intolerance, whereas among FK 506 treated patients 30% are frank diabetic and 40% have impaired tolerance [3]; similar features have been observed by other teams [4]. Studies comparing side effects of FK 506 and cyclosporine have also shown that calcineurin inhibitors induce diabetes or hyperglycemia (respectively 4% and 19%) and FK 506 appears to be more toxic in this regard [5, 6]. It is interesting to note that the use of FK 506 in pancreas transplantation has not induced post-transplantation diabetic states in initial studies.

Mycophenolate mofetil has not been shown to induce of favor post-transplantation hyperglycemic states.

Rapamycin is the latest immunophiline ligand. It shares a same cellular binding protein with FK 506, but its toxicity is different. Diabetes has been observed in rodents with this drug. So far, no toxicity in humans regarding glucose tolerance has been seen.

Monoclonal or polyclonal antibodies have not demonstrated a toxic effect for pancreatic β cells in organ transplantation. Their wide use has probably lowered the rate of post-operative acute rejection episodes, thus lowering the need for steroids.

How to minimize the diabetogenic effect of immunosuppressive drugs?

The use of low dose steroid regimens and steroid withdrawal has focused the interest of a number of transplantation centers. Steroid withdrawal could be of great interest in some categories of patients, such as those with high body mass index or the elderly, who are at particular risk for onset of diabetes after transplantation. It could also be essential for islet cells transplantation [7]. Steroid withdrawal has been attempted either early after renal or liver transplantation or after several months post transplantation [8]. In most clinical trials withdrawal of steroids is possible in nearly 80% of cases [9]; steroids have to be reintroduced for acute rejection in 20–25% of cases. However, creatinine levels tend to be slightly higher in patients not on steroids than in those receiving steroids [8–10]. Metabolic and clinical studies show that steroid-induced diabetes is reversed in three of four patients following steroid withdrawal [11], and glycated hemoglobin, lipid levels and hypertension are improved after steroid withdrawal. New powerful associations with Mycophenolate and FK 506 may help in the future to lower or even suppress steroid with less risks of rejection.

Switch to cyclosporine in patients with FK-induced diabetes has been successful. However some studies have shown that FK-induced diabetes is transient and essentially related to the dose of steroid given to the patients, lowering the dose of FK may also help reverse diabetes [12]. In some groups of patients above 60 years of age with high risk of onset of diabetes some teams have suggested withdrawal of calcineurin inhibitors [13]. This is justified by the increased risk of cardiovascular complications in this category of patient treated with steroids and calcineurin inhibitors.

Gene therapy-induced tolerance may, in the future enhance graft survival and lower the necessity of using diabetogenic drugs.

Conclusion

Some of the potent drugs used in transplantation demonstrate a diabetogenic effect. Steroid withdrawal is probably the first step to lower the diabetogenic effect of the immunosuppression.

References

1. Flanagan WH, Corthesy B, Bram RJ, Crabtree GR. Nuclear association of a T cell transcription factor blocked by FK 506 and cyclosporin A. Nature. 1991; 352: 803–807.
2. Isoniemi H. Renal Allograft Immunosuppression. Glucose intolerance occurring in different immunosuppressive treatments. Clin. Transplant. 1991; 5: 268–272.
3. Krentz AJ, Dousset B, Mayer D et al. Metabolic effects of cyclosporin and FK 506 in liver transplant recipients. Diabetes. 1993; 42: 1753–1759.
4. Jindal RM, Popescu I, Schwart ME, Emre S, Boccagni P, Miller CM. Diabetogenicity of FK versus cyclosporine in liver transplant recipients. Transplantation. 1994; 58: 370–372.
5. Pirsh JD, Miller J, Deierhoi MH, Vincenti F, Filo RS. A comparison of tacrolimus (FK 506) and cyclosporine for immunosuppression after cadaveric renal transplantation FK 506 Kidney Transplant Study Group. Transplantation. 1997; 63: 977–983.
6. Mayer AD, Dmitrewski J, Squifflet JP et al. Multicenter randomized trial comparing tacrolimus (FK 506) and cyclosporine in the prevention of renal allograft rejection: A report of the European Tacrolimus Multicenter Renal Study Group. Transplantation. 1997; 64: 436–443.
7. Sutherland D, Gruessner Gores P. Pancreas and islet cell transplantation. Transplant. Immunol. 1995; 147–160.
8. Fabrega AJ, Cohan J, Meslar P, Pollak R. Effect of steroid withdrawal on long term renal allograft recipients with post transplantation diabetes. Surgery. 1994; 116: 792–797.
9. Hollander AA, Hene RJ, Hermans J, Van Der Houde FJ. Late prednisone withdrawal in kidney transplanted patients. A randomized study. J. Am Soc. Nephrol. 1997; 8: 294–301.
10. Ratcliffe PJ, Dudley CR, Higgins RM, Firth JD, Morris PJ. Randomized controlled trial of steroid withdrawal in renal transplant patients receiving triple immunosuppression. Lancet. 1996; 348: 643–648.
11. Stegall MD, Wachs ME, Everson G, Steinberg T, Bilir B, Shrestha R, Karrer F, Kam I. Predisone withdrawal 14 days after liver transplantation with Mycophenolate. Transplantation. 1997; 64: 1755–1760.
12. Shapiro R, Scantlabury VP, Jordan ML, Starzl TE. Reversibility of tacrolimus induced posttransplant diabetes: an illustrative case and review of the literature. Transplant. Proc. 1997; 29: 2737–2738.
13. Zanker B, Schneebeeberger H, Rothenpieler U et al. Mucophenolate mofetil-based, cyclosporine-free induction and maintenance immunosuppression. Transplantation. 1998; 66: 44–49.

13. Can we minimize long-term side effects of immunosuppressive drugs on lipid metabolism?

Z. A. MASSY

Introduction

Hyperlipidemia (also referred to as dyslipidemia) is common after solid organ transplantation. It has been reported in more than 60% of heart [1], kidney [2, 3], and lung transplant recipients [4], as well as in more than 30% of liver transplant recipients [5, 6].

Hyperlipidemia is one of the most common causes of the increased cardiovascular morbidity and mortality observed among long-term survivors of renal transplantation [3, 7]. It has also been correlated with an increased risk for peripheral vascular disease in cardiac transplant recipients [8–10], and has been associated with allograft vasculopathy in cardiac [11, 12] and in renal transplantation [7, 13]. It should be noted that the relationship of hyperlipidemia to post-transplant cardiovascular disease and to allograft vasculopathy in other solid organ transplantation is not clearly defined [14, 15].

Immunosuppressive therapy, particularly corticosteroids, cyclosporine A and, recently, rapamycin, has been identified as an important factor involved in the genesis of post-transplant hyperlipidemia [7, 16, 17]. Although the relative contribution of immunosuppressive therapy to post-transplant hyperlipidemia is not fully clarified, it is clear that it is related to immunosuppressive therapy in a dose-dependent fashion [7, 17]. Taking into consideration the potential risk of post-transplantation hyperlipidemia, it is reasonable to assume that strategies to minimize the effects of immunosuppressive therapy on lipid metabolism and/or on its cardiovascular consequences could be helpful in reducing cardiovascular morbidity and mortality and allograft vasculopathy in solid organ transplant recipients. In this review, I will focus on such therapeutic options.

Modulation of immunosuppressive therapy

The ideal immunosuppressive therapy does not exist. However, modulation of existing regimens to improve the long-term side effects of immunosuppressive therapy, including hyperlipidemia, without affecting allograft survival is feasible. One strategy to reduce hyperlipidemia is to modify the dosage, or even withdraw the immunosuppressive drug implicated in its genesis. Changing to

P. Cochat et al. (eds.), Immunosuppression under Trial, 105–109
©1999 Kluwer Academic Publishers.

alternate-day prednisone administration can be effective in lowering lipid levels [18], although not everyone has obtained success with this strategy [19, 20]. Complete corticosteroid withdrawal, while maintaining the transplant recipients on cyclosporine A and azathioprine can also be effective in reducing hyperlipidemia [21–25]. It should be noted that not all patients may benefit from such an approach, and caution is needed with regard to the long-term outcome [22–25]. However, the recent use of mycophenolate mofetil in association with cyclosporine A may widen the possibility of corticosteroid withdrawal with increased success [26]. In some renal transplant recipients cyclosporine A can be withdrawn in the late post-transplant period, and hyperlipidemia can be improved as a result [27]. Circumstantial data suggest that the success of cyclosporine A withdrawal is influenced by the number of HLA mismatches [28, 29]. Thus better matching may reduce hyperlipidemia and other complications, by reducing the requirements for long-term immunosuppressive therapy with high doses of toxic medications.

A second strategy for reducing hyperlipidemia consists of substituting corticosteroids or cyclosporine A by the newer immunosuppressive agents that have fewer adverse effects on lipid metabolism. Recent data suggest that it may be possible to replace prednisone with deflazacort (an alternative corticosteroid) which has fewer effects on blood lipids [30]. Moreover, conversion from cyclosporine A to tacrolimus in hyperlipemic renal transplant recipients was associated with a moderate reduction in low density lipoprotein [31]. In a recent small study, hyperlipidemia was improved after conversion from cyclosporine A and azathioprine to mycophenolate mofetil in six renal transplant recipients [32]. These studies are small, but if the results are confirmed by large controlled studies, they offer promise of a new strategy to modulate immunosuppressive therapy in order to improve hyperlipidemia.

Lipid lowering therapies

Since the optimization of immunosuppressive regimens corrects only moderately the levels of lipids in solid organ transplant recipients, it is clear that lipid lowering therapies are necessary in such patients. Diet and lipid lowering drugs are the two arms of such a strategy. However, dietary intervention has no consistent effects on post-transplant hyperlipidemia [2, 33], and the additional use of lipid lowering drugs is probably needed. Among lipid lowering drugs, 3-hydroxy-3-methyl-glutaryl coenzyme A (HMG-CoA) reductase inhibitors, and fibric acid derivatives are the most effective agents [2, 33–37]. Since blood levels of HMG-CoA reductase inhibitors have been shown to be high under cyclosporine and tacrolimus treatment [38], it is necessary to halve the doses of HMG-CoA reductase inhibitors in solid organ transplant recipients receiving such treatment. Adjusted doses of fibric acid derivatives, particularly gemfibrozil, are also necessary given the reduced renal function in some patients [39, 40]. Two recent studies have demonstrated that the use of HMG-CoA reductase inhibitors after cardiac transplantation has beneficial effects, not only on lipid abnormalities, but also on the incidence of acute rejection and coronary vasculopathy [41, 42]. A similar study after kidney transplantation confirmed these findings concerning the incidence of acute rejection, but failed to demonstrate any effect on 1-year renal function [43]. Thus, the reduction of cardiovascular morbidity and mortality and allograft vasculopathy by lipid lowering drugs has not yet been demonstrated in renal transplant recipients. However, a large, prospective, randomized, European study on the effects of fluvastatin on cardiovascular death and the development of chronic renal allograft rejection is now in progress. In the meantime, the use of adequate approaches to correct hyperlipidemia in renal transplant recipients who have cardiovascular disease or multiple risk factors for cardiovascular disease seems appropriate. These interventions may also influence the development of allograft vasculopathy as shown in cardiac transplant recipients [41, 42].

Conclusions

Hyperlipidemia is common after solid organ transplantation, and it is associated with post-transplant cardiovascular disease and allograft vasculopathy. Immunosuppressive therapy is one of the principal factors involved in post-transplant hyperlipidemia. Optimization of immunosuppressive regimens compatible with prolonged allograft survival, together with the use of lipid lowering therapies, will help minimize post-transplant hyperlipidemia and its potential harmful consequences.

References

1. Miller LW, Schlant RC, Kobashigawa J, Kubo S, Renlund DG. 24th Bethesda conference: cardiac transplantation. Task Force 5: complications. J. Am. Coll. Cardiol. 1993; 22: 41–54.
2. Massy ZA, Ma JZ, Louis TA, Kasiske BL. Lipid-lowering therapy in patients with renal disease. Kidney Int. 1995; 48: 188–198.
3. Kasiske BL. Hyperlipidemia in patients with chronic renal disease. Am. J. Kidney Dis. 1998; 32: S142–S156.
4. Kesten S, Mayne L, Scavuzzo M, Maurer J. Lack of left ventricular dysfunction associated with sustained exposure to hyperlipidemia following lung transplantation. Chest. 1997; 112: 931–936.
5. Stegall MD, Everson G, Schroter G, Bilir B, Karrer F, Kam I. Metabolic complications after liver transplantation. Transplantation. 1995; 60: 1057–1060.
6. Mathe D, Adam R, Malmendier C et al. Prevalence of dyslipidemia in liver transplant recipients. Transplantation. 1992; 54: 167–170.
7. Massy A, Kasiske BL. Post-transplant hyperlipidemia: mechanisms and management. J. Am. Soc. Nephrol. 1996; 7: 971–977.
8. Bull DA, Hunter GC, Copeland JG et al. Peripheral vascular disease in heart transplant recipients. J. Vasc. Surg. 1992; 16: 546–553.
9. Julia P, Amrein C, Ghalayini B et al. Peripheral vascular involvement in heart transplant patients. Ann. Vasc. Surg. 1994; 8: 266–270.
10. Erdoes LS, Hunter GC, Venerus BJ et al. Prospective evaluation of peripheral vascular disease in heart transplant recipients. J. Vasc. Surg. 1995; 22: 434–442.

11. McManus BM, Horley KJ, Wilson JE et al. Prominence of coronary arterial wall lipids in human heart allografts. Implications for pathogenesis of allograft arteriopathy. Am. J. Pathol. 1995; 147: 293–308.
12. Billingham ME. Pathology and etiology of chronic rejection of the heart. Clin. Transplant. 1994; 8: 289–292.
13. Vollmer E, Bosse A, Bögeholz J et al. Apolipoproteins and immunohistological differentiation of cells in the arterial wall of kidneys in transplant arteriopathy. Morphological parallels with atherosclerosis. Pathol. Res. Pract. 1991; 187: 957–962.
14. Morrissey PE, Shaffer D, Monaco AP, Conway P, Madras PN. Peripheral vascular disease after kidney-pancreas transplantation in diabetic patients with end-stage renal disease. Arch. Surg. 1997; 132: 358–361.
15. Dec GW, Kondo N, Farrell ML, Dienstag JL, Cosimi AB, Semigran MJ. Cardiovascular complications following liver transplantation. Clin. Transplant. 1995; 9: 463–471.
16. Butman SM. Hyperlipidemia after cardiac transplantation: be aware and possibly wary of drug therapy for lowering of serum lipids. Am. Heart. J. 1991; 121: 1585–1590.
17. Brattström C, Wilczek H, Tydén G, Böttiger Y, Säwe J, Groth CG. Hyperlipidemia in renal transplant recipients treated with sirolimus (rapamycin). Transplantation. 1998; 65: 1272–1274.
18. Curtis JJ, Galla JH, Woodford SY, Lucas BA, Luke RG. Effect of alternate-day prednisone on plasma lipids in renal transplant recipients. Kidney Int. 1982; 22: 42–47.
19. Drukker A, Turner C, Start K et al. Hyperlipidemia after renal transplantation in children on alternate day corticosteroid therapy. Clin. Nephrol. 1986; 26: 140–145.
20. Sinclair NR. Low-dose steroid therapy in cyclosporine-treated renal transplant recipients with well-functioning grafts. The Canadian Multicentre Transplant Study Group [see comments]. CMAJ. 1992; 147: 645–657.
21. Hricik DE, Bartucci MR, Mayes JT, Schulak JA. The effects of steroid withdrawal on the lipoprotein profiles of cyclosporine-treated kidney and kidney–pancreas transplant recipients. Transplantation. 1992; 54: 868–871.
22. Hollander AA, Hene RJ, Hermans J, Van Es LA, van der Woude FJ. Late prednisone withdrawal in cyclosporine-treated kidney transplant patients: a randomized study. J. Am. Soc. Nephrol. 1997; 8: 294–301.
23. Renlund DG, Bristow MR, Crandall BG et al. Hypercholesterolemia after heart transplantation: amelioration by corticosteroid-free maintenance immunosuppression. J. Heart. Transplant. 1989; 8: 214–219; discussion 219–220.
24. Keogh A, Macdonald P, Harvison A, Richens D, Mundy J, Spratt P. Initial steroid-free versus steroid-based maintenance therapy and steroid withdrawal after heart transplantation: two views of the steroid question. J. Heart. Lung Transplant. 1992; 11: 421–427.
25. Ratcliffe PJ, Dudley CRK, Higgins RM, Firth JD, Smith B, Morris J. Randomised controlled trial of steroid withdrawal in renal transplant recipients receiving triple immunosuppression. Lancet. 1996; 348: 643–648.
26. Birkeland SA. Steroid-free immunosuppression after kidney transplantation with antithymocyte globulin induction and cyclosporine and mycophenolate mofetil maintenance therapy. Transplantation. 1998; 66: 1207–1210.
27. Sutherland F, Burgess E, Klassen J, Buckle S, Paul LC. Post-transplant conversion from cyclosporin to azathioprine: effect on cardiovascular risk profile. Transplant. Int. 1993; 6: 129–132.
28. Heim-Duthoy KL, Chitwood KK, Tortorice KL, Massy ZA, Kasiske BL. Elective cyclosporine withdrawal 1 year after renal transplantation. Am. J. Kidney. Dis. 1994; 24: 846–853.
29. Hollander AAMJ, van Saase JLCM, Kootte AMM et al. Beneficial effects of conversion from cyclosporine to azathioprine after kidney transplantation. Lancet. 1995; 345: 610–614.
30. Lippuner K, Casez JP, Horber FF, Jaeger P. Effects of deflazacort versus prednisone on bone mass, body composition, and lipid profile: a randomized, double blind study in kidney transplant patients. J. Clin. Endocrinol. Metab. 1998; 83: 3795–3802.
31. McCune TR, Thacker LRI, Peters TG et al. Effects of tacrolimus on hyperlipidemia after

successful renal transplantation. Transplantation. 1998; 65: 87–92.

32. Ducloux D, Fournier V, Bresson-Vautrin C et al. Mycophenolate mofetil in renal transplant recipients with cyclosporine-associated nephrotoxicity: a preliminary report. Transplantation. 1998; 65: 1504–1506.

33. Ballantyne CM, Radovancevic B, Farmer JA et al. Hyperlipidemia after heart transplantation: report of a 6-year experience, with treatment recommendations. J. Am. Coll. Cardiol. 1992; 19: 1315–1321.

34. Stapleton DD, Mehra MR, Dumas D et al. Lipid-lowering therapy and long-term survival in heart transplantation. Am. J. Cardiol. 1997; 80: 802–805.

35. Zambrana JL, Velasco F, Castro P et al. Comparison of bezafibrate versus lovastatin for lowering plasma insulin, fibrinogen, plasminogen activator inhibitor-1 concentrations in hyperlipemic heart transplant patients. Am. J. Cardiol. 1997; 80: 836–840.

36. Imagawa DK, Dawson III S, Holt CD et al. Hyperlipidemia after liver transplantation. Transplantation. 1996; 62: 934–942.

37. Al'Halawani MH, Larsen JL, Miller S, Frisbie K, Taylor RJ, Stratta RJ. Pravastatin reduces serum cholesterol and low density lipoprotein concentrations following pancreas transplantation. Transplantation. 1994; 58: 1204–1209.

38. Christians U, Jacobsen W, Floren LC. Metabolism and drug interactions of 3-hydroxy-3-methylglutaryl coenzyme A reductase inhibitors in transplant patients: Are the statins mechanistically similar? Pharmacol. Ther. 1998; 80: 1–34.

39. Chan TM, Cheng IKP, Tam SCF. Hyperlipidemia after renal transplantation: treatment with gemfibrozil. Nephron. 1994; 67: 317–321.

40. Fuhrer JA, Montandon A, Descoeudres C, Jaeger P, Horber FF. Impact of time-interval after transplantation and therapy with fibrates on serum cholesterol levels in renal transplant patients. Clin. Nephrol. 1993; 39: 265–271.

41. Kobashigawa JA, Katznelson S, Laks H et al. Effect of pravastatin on outcomes after cardiac transplantation. N. Engl. J. Med. 1995; 333: 621–627.

42. Wenke K, Meiser BM, Thiery J et al. Simvastatin reduces graft vessel disease and mortality after heart transplantation – a four-year randomized trial. Circulation. 1997; 96: 1398–1402.

43. Katznelson S, Wilkinson AH, Kobashigawa JA et al. The effect of pravastatin on acute rejection after kidney transplantation – a pilot study. Transplantation. 1996; 61: 1469–1474.

14. Can we minimize the long-term side effects of immunosuppressive drugs in pediatric patients?

B. TÖNSHOFF, O. MEHLS and L. WEBER

Introduction

Renal transplantation is the treatment of choice for end-stage renal disease in children, leading to substantial improvement in the quality of life. However, despite a significant improvement in short-term results, important long-term problems remain unsolved. Allograft half-life has only slightly improved in pediatric renal transplant recipients during the last decade due to the lack of effective treatment for chronic rejection, frequent recipient non-compliance, particularly in adolescence, and nephrotoxicity of the immunosuppressive calcineurin inhibitors cyclosporine A and tacrolimus. Therefore, a pediatric renal graft recipient is likely to need several retransplantations during his life. Furthermore, the immunosuppressive drugs used today have potentially serious side effects, including infection, nephrotoxicity and *de novo* malignancy. These topics are particularly relevant for children who are likely to receive immuno-suppressive therapy for several decades. The biological differences between an adult and a growing and developing pediatric transplant recipient also have to be taken into account. It is important, therefore, to develop immunosup-pressive protocols that are adjusted to the specific needs of a growing child.

In the last few years, new and more efficient immunosuppressive drugs have emerged on the market and may possibly contribute to overcoming chronic rejection. However, specific tolerance, the holy grail of organ transplantation, is not likely to be achieved during the next decade. Accordingly, long-term side effects of immunosuppressive drugs will become even more important as more patients are treated for increasingly longer periods of time. It is important, therefore, to understand the properties of these new drugs in children, aiming at optimal graft survival but also at avoiding unnecessary adverse effects. This article will review some important long-term side effects of immunosuppressive drugs in pediatric patients, such as nephrotoxicity, malignancy, and growth inhibition, and discuss potential strategies to minimize their toxicity.

Nephrotoxicity of cyclosporine A and tacrolimus

Cyclosporine A and tacrolimus have both a high nephrotoxic potential.

P. Cochat et al. (eds.), Immunosuppression under Trial, 111–121
©1999 Kluwer Academic Publishers.

Cyclosporine nephrotoxicity is manifested both as acute azotemia, which is largely reversible after reducing the dose, or as chronic progressive renal disease, which is usually irreversible.

The acute nephrotoxicity caused by cyclosporine A and tacrolimus is due to the vasoconstrictive effects of the drugs on the afferent arterioles, leading to a decrease in glomerular filtration rate (GFR) and renal plasma flow (RPF) [1]. This increase in vascular resistance is reflected clinically by an elevated plasma creatinine concentration and hypertension. Cyclosporine-induced renal vasocontriction can cause delayed recovery from early acute tubular necrosis and, in severe cases, primary non-function. These complications are most likely to occur with prolonged ischemia time and high cyclosporine doses, but even patients with therapeutic trough levels may show signs of nephrotoxicity [2]. Acute cyclosporine nephrotoxicity is usually reversible with reduction or cessation of therapy. Tubular effects of cyclosporine A may manifest as hyperkalemia due to decreased distal nephron K^+ secretion [3], hyperuricemia due to increased proximal tubular uric acid reabsorption [4], renal Mg^{2+} wasting, metabolic acidosis by impairment of acid excretion, hypophosphatemia due to urinary phosphate wasting and decreased urinary concentrating capacity.

Chronic cyclosporine nephrotoxicity is manifested by renal insufficiency due to glomerular and vascular disease, abnormalities in tubular function and an increase in blood pressure [5]. Although cyclosporine A has had a major impact on renal allograft survival by reducing graft loss due to acute rejection, it does not affect the rate at which renal allografts are lost to chronic rejection. Thus, the half-lives of renal allografts in the cyclosporine era are not very different from those seen before cyclosporine was available [6]. One possible explanation for this observation is that cyclosporine itself contributes to chronic nephropathy leading to allograft dysfunction and ultimate graft loss.

Renal histology in established chronic cyclosporine A nephrotoxicity reveals an obliterative arteriolopathy, suggesting primary endothelial damage, ischemic collapse or scarring of the glomeruli, vacuolization of the tubules, and focal areas of tubular atrophy and interstitial fibrosis. These changes seem to occur earlier with higher doses of cyclosporine A [7], although they are seen also with low-dose regimes.

Both short- and long-term studies in liver transplant recipients suggest that tacrolimus is at least as nephrotoxic as cyclosporine A. Long-term trials have found a similar incidence of early acute renal failure, late hypertension and late renal insufficiency, although the latter may be somewhat more prevalent with tacrolimus [8–10]. Tacrolimus can also cause hyperkalemia, hyperuricemia and, rarely, hemolytic-uremic syndrome [8, 11].

Strategies to avoid nephrotoxicity

Monitoring of kidney function is important in avoiding calcineurin inhibitor-associated nephrotoxicity. Serum creatinine is not a sensitive marker of GFR and when used alone it does not allow for detection of the early signs of nephrotoxicity. Occasional measurements of GFR by clearance methods and monitoring tubular parameters, such as potassium and uric acid, significantly increase drug safety. The reductions in RPF and GFR are correlated both with dose and with peak cyclosporine levels reached 2–4 hours after the oral dose [12]. Because young (preschool) children have a faster cyclosporine A metabolism, some centers give cyclosporine A to these children in three daily doses in order to avoid high and potentially toxic peak drug concentrations [13].

There is no general agreement on the optimal dose of cyclosporine A in pediatric renal transplantation. A recent report from the North American Pediatric Renal Transplant Cooperative Study (NAPRTCS) group suggests that a higher maintenance cyclosporine dose decreases the risk of graft failure in pediatric renal transplant recipients [14]: at 6 months after transplantation, the maintenance cyclosporine dose in 1103 living donor graft recipients, who retained graft function during the subsequent 6-month period, was 7.1 mg/kg per day, compared with 3.9 mg/kg per day in 28 patients who lost their graft in the subsequent 6-month period. For 1041 recipients of cadaver donor grafts who retained graft function for 12 months after transplantation, the 6-month maintenance cyclosporine dose was 7.4 mg/kg per day, compared with 5.4 mg/kg per day in 59 patients whose graft failed in the subsequent 6 months. In patients who did not have an acute rejection episode during the 12 months after transplantation, the rate of subsequent late rejections was 22% for patients with a 12-month maintenance cyclosporine dose ≤ 4 mg/kg per day, and 16% for patients whose 12-month maintenance cyclosporine dose exceeded 8.6 mg/kg per day [14].

Severe cyclosporine toxicity has been rare at our center. We begin with a cyclosporine A dose of 10 mg/kg per day in the perioperative period, aiming at cyclosporine A whole blood trough levels (by RIA) at 100–170 ng/ml, and taper the dose after 3 months to trough levels of 70–140 ng/ml. We generally perform renal allograft biopsies in any patient with an unexplained elevation in the plasma creatinine concentration. A presumptive diagnosis of cyclosporine nephrotoxicity is made if there are no signs of acute rejection. In this setting, lowering of the cyclosporine A dose by 0.5–1 mg/kg per day leads to a reversal of renal dysfunction within a few days in patients with acute or subacute nephrotoxicity. In contrast, patients who have chronic rejection on renal biopsy may benefit from raising the dose of cyclosporine A, as the plasma creatinine concentration may stabilize or even decrease. We use the calcium channel inhibitor diltiazem in the first 2 weeks after transplantation in order to prevent the acute renal vasoconstriction induced by cyclosporine A. A general renoprotective effect of calcium channel inhibitors in the long-term has not yet been proven [15, 16].

In patients with established chronic cyclosporine A nephrotoxicity, the replacement of cyclosporine A with non-nephrotoxic immunosuppressive agents may ameliorate renal dysfunction. In one study, 10 patients with biopsy-verified cyclosporine nephrotoxicity were switched from an immunosuppressive regimen of cyclosporine and prednisone to dual therapy with mycophenolate mofetil and prednisone [17]. The dose of prednisone was maintained, cyclosporine was withdrawn over 6 weeks, and mycophenolate mofetil was begun at 2 g/day. At 11 months, there was a significant improvement in the creatinine clearance (55 versus 46 ml/min per 1.73 m^2) with no episodes of acute rejection. Another study of six patients with biopsy-proven cyclosporine nephrotoxicity found that the conversion from a cyclosporine–azathioprine to a mycophenolate mofetil based regimen lowered the mean serum creatinine concentration of from 225 to 159 μmol/l at one year [18]. No episode of acute rejections was observed. These preliminary observations indicate that a cyclosporine-free mycophenolate mofetil-based regimen can be applied in patients with cyclosporine toxicity, but the long-term efficacy of this regimen requires further evaluation.

Malignancy

The chronic use of maintenance immunosuppressive agents to prevent allograft rejection increases the long-term risk of malignancy. In adult renal transplant recipients, the relative overall cancer risk is 3.4 times higher than that in the general population [19]; the overall incidence has been reported to range from 4% to 18%, with a mean of 6% [20]. a variety of neoplasms occur with increased frequency in transplant recipients, including squamous cell carcinomas of the skin, non-Hodgkin's lymphoma, Kaposi's sarcoma, in situ carcinomas of the uterine cervix, carcinomas of the vulva and perineum, renal carcinoma, hepatobiliary carcinomas, and a variety of sarcomas [21]. In contrast, the incidence of many of the most common tumors in the general population, such as lung, prostate, colon and invasive uterine carcinomas, is not increased [22].

There are few data on the incidence of malignancy in pediatric renal transplant recipients. In the NAPRTCS registry data, 16 malignancies were identified in 2037 recipients over a 5-year period [23]. Eleven of these were lymphoid organ (five cases of lymphoproliferative disorder, four cases of lymphoma and two cases of immunoblastic carcinomas). Malignancies are still a relatively rare cause of death in pediatric renal transplant recipients: in an analysis of 2457 patients from the NAPRTCS registry who were followed for 5481 patient–years after transplantation 136 deaths were observed with an average annual rate of 24.8 deaths per 1000 patient–years. Death resulted primarily from infection (40%), cardiovascular causes (21%), hemorrhage (12%), and malignancies (7%) [24].

Anti-lymphocyte therapy, such as OKT3 or anti-lymphocyte serum, specifically predisposes to post-transplant lymphoproliferative disorders which are induced by Epstein-Barr virus. With this exception, there is no evidence that a particular immunosuppressive agent causes a specific type of malignancy. Rather, it is the overall level of immunosuppression that the patient has received and continues to receive that increases the risk of post-transplant malignancy. This relationship explains why lymphoproliferative disorders, for example, are more common in recipients of solid, non-renal organs such as the heart [25]. These patients receive more aggressive anti-rejection therapy, since loss of such organs would result in death while the renal transplant recipient can return to dialysis. The concept that the degree of immunosuppression determines the risk to develop malignancy is supported by a recent randomized study in adults comparing a low-dose (trough whole blood concentrations 75–125 ng/ml) and a standard (150–250 ng/ml) cyclosporine A regimen [26]. At 66 months' follow-up, the two groups were similar in mean serum creatinine and creatinine clearance. Nine of 116 patients in the low-dose group and one of 115 in the normal-dose group had symptoms of rejection ($p < 0.02$). There was no difference between the two groups in survival (95 versus 92%) or graft survival (89 versus 82%; $p = 0.17$) at 6 years, but of 60 patients who developed cancer, 37 were in the standard group and 23 in the low-dose group ($p < 0.034$) [26]. Hence, the design of long-term maintenance protocols for transplant recipients based on powerful immunosuppressive combinations should take these potential risks into account.

The lymphoproliferative disorder is currently a focus of discussion in pediatric transplantation. There are some data that it may occur five to six times more often in children than in adults [27], and may be fatal, although cases of spontaneous involution occur after withdrawal of immunosuppression. The full extent of the problem of malignancy will become evident during the coming decades when a large number of pediatric recipients have been followed up over a sufficiently long time.

Cancer in the renal transplant recipient is rarely a consequence of transmission from the donor [28, 29]. A variety of malignancies has been transmitted, including cancer of the lung, breast, colon, rectum and kidney. In one review, malignancy developed in 78 of 142 (45%) of patients who received a cadaver graft from a donor subsequently found to have a tumor [29].

Prophylaxis and treatment of malignancy

An approach to treatment of post-transplant malignancies should begin with preventive measures. In particular, excess immunosuppression or repeated exposure to anti-lymphocyte antibodies should be avoided. With regard to skin cancers, sun exposure should be limited with either avoidance or protective sunscreens and clothing. Patients should be examined regularly and any premalignant lesions should be treated. Metabolites of azathioprine sensitize the skin to sunlight and may increase the risk of local malignancy [30].

There are two malignancies in which reduction in or cessation of immunosuppressive therapy may result in regression of the tumor: lymphoma and Kaposi's sarcoma, in which reducing the cyclosporine exposure may be particularly important [22]. This approach is useful primarily in renal transplantation, since loss of the graft to rejection is not a fatal event. Alpha interferon has also been used successfully in patients with Kaposi's sarcoma, although there is a risk of precipitating acute rejection [31].

Growth failure

Successful renal transplantation reverses the uremic milieu and should theoretically permit normal growth hormone (GH) secretion and function. Persistent growth failure in this setting is primarily due to reduced graft function and glucocorticoid therapy. Pharmacological doses of glucocorticoids interfere at different levels with the integrity of the somatotropic hormone axis. The majority of patients on chronic corticosteroid medication present overt GH hyposecretion, apparently due to enhancement of hypothalamic somato-statin release [32]. Glucocorticoids also inhibit insulin-like growth factor (IGF) bioactivity by the induction of IGF inhibitors and stimulate the production of certain IGF binding proteins. In addition, glucocorticoids inhibit growth directly at the tissue level by suppressing local growth factors and skeletal tissue matrix production [32]. The cumulative amount of glucocorticoids is certainly a determinant of the growth rates achieved post-transplantation. The introduction of cyclosporine A for pediatric renal transplant recipients in 1984 allowed a reduction in the dose of the concomitant glucocorticoid medication. However, improved growth rates were only reported by some investigators [33]. It also appears that final height has not been consistently improved by the introduction of cyclosporine A in comparison with conventional immunosuppression.

Another determinant of growth post-transplant is the function of the renal graft. In a report from the NAPRTCS registry following 300 children with a functioning graft over 2 years, an increase in the serum creatinine concentration by 1.0 mg/dl was associated with a decrease in height SD score of 0.17 /p year [34]. The age of the recipient at time of transplantation, and consequently the residual growth potential, also influences the degree of growth improvement. In the experience of the NAPRTCS registry, catch-up growth, as defined as a gain of relative height of at least 1 SD in 2 years, occurred in 50% of the group aged 0–1 year, 25% of the group aged 2–5 years, 16% of the group aged 6–12 years, and 6% of the group aged 13–17 years. Similar unfavorable results were reported by Hokken-Koelega [35], who observed in a retrospective analysis of 70 prepubertal children during the first 2 years after renal transplantation an increment in height SD of less than 0.5 SD for 70% of the study population. Patients with the most severe growth retardation at transplantation appeared to have the most pronounced growth spurt after transplantation, but even they never had complete catch-up growth. These data show that in the first years post-transplant, when renal function is still stable, height acceleration does not occur in most of the children over the age of 6 years, and alternative strategies are necessary to improve the quality of life in these children.

Strategies for optimization of growth post-transplant – steroid reduction or withdrawal

The mode of administration of glucocorticoids appears to be related to their growth-depressing properties, with an alternate-day regimen being more favorable than a daily dose. Broyer et al. [36] reported the first prospective controlled study involving 35 patients with a graft function > 50 ml/min per 1.73 m^2 treated either with daily prednisone, 0.25 mg/kg per day, or on an alternate-day regimen with the same cumulative steroid dosage. In prepubertal children on alternate-day therapy, a marked increase in height of 0.60 ± 0.31 SD during the first treatment year was observed compared with prepubertal children on daily treatment (change in height per year 0.04 ± 0.31 SD). No acute rejection episode in the alternate-day group occurred. In a retrospective analysis of 2001 patients from the NAPRTCS, 16.8% of pediatric renal transplant recipients were receiving alternate-day steroids [37]. During the first 2 years after transplantation, the mean change in height SD was significantly greater in those on alternate-day dosing (+0.50 ± 0.06 SD) than in those on daily dosing (+0.10 ± 0.03 SD) without compromising allograft survival or function.

Only a few medical centers have studied the effect of glucocorticoid withdrawal on growth and graft function. In a selected group of patients with stable graft function Klare et al. [38] observed a mean increase in relative height of 0.8 ± 0.3 SD in the first year and 0.3 ± 0.2 SD in the second year after renal transplantation in response to steroid withdrawal in 12 children with a serum creatinine below 2.0 mg/dl. These data indicate that, at least in children with only slightly reduced graft function, cessation of glucocorticoids can induce catch-up growth. However, this regimen certainly increases the risk of graft rejection with a reported incidence of 39% as summarized experience from the literature [39]. To reduce the risk of graft rejection, the patient has to be maintained on higher doses of cyclosporine which, on the other hand, increases the risk of cyclosporine nephrotoxicity. Currently, it does therefore not seem justified to withdraw steroids on a protocol basis in patients on conventional immunosuppressive drugs.

The strategy of steroid withdrawal may be more successful in the future, because new and more potent drugs, such as tacrolimus and mycophenolate mofetil, are now available for maintenance immunosuppressive therapy. In the Pittsburgh experience, 24 of 39 children (62%) on tacrolimus therapy could be successfully withdrawn from steroids [40]. Improved growth was seen, particularly in pre-adolescent children off steroids with a mean increase of relative height from –2.54 ± 1.27 SD at transplant to –0.55 ± 2.03 SD after 1 year of treatment. However, the use of tacrolimus instead of cyclosporine A as a primary immunosuppressive agent is still under debate, because the greater efficacy of tacrolimus must be weighed against the higher incidence of side-effects.

Preliminary evidence in adult renal transplant recipients indicates that glucocorticoids can safely be withdrawn from the immunosuppressive regimen in stable patients on cyclosporine A and mycophenolate mofetil [41]. In an open pilot study, steroids were withdrawn from 26 adult cadaveric kidney transplant recipients. Corticosteroids were discontinued between 4 and 30 (mean 17) months after transplantation, and steroid-free follow-up ranged from 7 to 18 (mean 10) months. Mean cyclosporine A doses, cyclosporine A blood levels, and serum creatinine at the time of steroid withdrawal and at last patient visit after cessation of steroids were 4.2 ± 1.2 mg/kg per day and 3.0 ± 0.8 mg/kg per day ($p < 0.001$), 170 ± 53 ng/ml and 113 ± 34 ng/ml ($p < 0.001$), and 133 ± 36 μmol/l and 130 μmol/l, respectively. No rejection episodes occurred after steroid withdrawal [41].

Concomitant anabolic treatment with recombinant human growth hormone

If catch-up growth cannot be achieved by an alternate-day steroid regime and if discontinuation of steroids is an intolerable risk for graft survival recombinant human growth hormone (rhGH) therapy may be initiated [33]. However, not all safety aspects of rhGH in this group of children have been sufficiently studied, in particular the effect of rhGH on graft function. As a result, the therapeutic use of rhGH in children after transplantation should be restricted to clinical trials.

Exogenous GH reverses the catabolic and growth-depressing effects of glucocorticoids in both experimental and clinical settings [42]. In particular, rhGH can counteract the interference of pharmacological doses of glucocorticoids with the integrity of the GH/IGF axis. There are two rationales for rhGH administration in short children with renal transplants: (1) rhGH treatment can be considered as substitution therapy in individuals with glucocorticoid-induced GH hyposecretion. (2) rhGH is able to restore IGF bioactivity in children who secrete normal amounts of GH but have decreased biologically available IGF [43].

The short-term growth responses to rhGH has been documented in a number of open-labeled prospective studies with observation periods of 1–3 years [42]. Height velocity in the first treatment year in prepubertal children can be doubled by rhGH treatment. The growth-promoting effect of rhGH moderately declines in the second and third treatment year [43], as observed in rhGH trials for other treatment indications. However, because the natural course of growth in children post-transplantation tends to progressively decelerate, even modest improvement in growth rates, if sustained, can result in normalization of longitudinal growth. In our experience with children who remained prepubertal during the observation period, three of seven patients achieved a normal relative height after 2 years of treatment [43].

Data from the first large randomized study on rhGH treatment in children after kidney transplantation have been reported recently [44]. In the first year, height velocity was significantly increased by rhGH, 7.7 cm in the treated group versus 4.6 cm in the control group. During the subsequent years of treatment, a decrease in growth velocity was noted compared with the first year data, but growth rates remained above the values obtained before treatment: 5.9 cm at 2 years, 5.5 cm at 3 years, and 5.2 cm at 4 years. The mean change in glomerular filtration rate did not differ between the treated and control groups during the first year of the study. In children with no or one rejection episode prior to GH (three patients in each group treated 27, control 25) had a new rejection episode during the first year of the trial. However, in children with a history of two or more rejections, six of the 17 treated patients had a new episode, but only one of the 12 control patients [44]. These data show that acute rejection episodes appear to be more frequent during rhGH administration in those patients who have a history of more than one episode. Close monitoring of graft function is therefore recommended. On the other hand, rhGH appears to be safe in immunologically low-risk patients with a history of one or less acute rejection episodes.

Summary

The issue of the choice of long-term immunosuppressive drug therapy in renal transplantation is unclear because we know so little of the pathogenesis of chronic allograft nephropathy. The assumption that much of late graft loss is an on-going immune response is widely questioned, and the practice of the long-term use of progressively more powerful immunosuppressive protocols may be potentially dangerous (e.g. risk of malignancy). While the necessity of some long-term immunosuppression is accepted as given, the choice of the protocol is unclear. A long-term immunosuppression protocol in pediatric renal transplant recipients has to take into account the biological differences between an adult and a growing and developing child. The currently used immunosuppressive protocols based on cyclosporine A and glucocorticoids have the frequent long-term side effects of nephrotoxicity, hypertension and growth inhibition. The long-term use of newer immunosuppressive drugs, such as mycophenolate mofetil, with no cyclosporine A or glucocorticoids has not been investigated in children. The lack of hypertension, lipid abnormalities, organ toxicity and growth-depressing effects may be a strong factor in favoring evaluation of this alternative in pediatric renal transplant recipients [45].

References

1. Mason J. The pathophysiology of Sandimmune (cyclosporine) in man and animals. Pediatr. Nephrol. 1990; 4: 554–574.
2. Novick AC, Ho-Hsieh H, Steinmuller DS et al. Detrimental effect of cyclosporine on initial function of cadaver renal allografts following extended preservation: Results of randomized prospective trial. Transplantation. 1986; 42: 154–158.
3. Laine J, Holmberg C. Renal and adrenal mechanisms in cyclosporine induced hyperkalemia after renal transplantation. Eur. J. Clin. Invest. 1995; 25: 670–676.
4. Laine J, Holmberg C. Mechanisms of hyperuricemia renal transplanted children. Nephron. 1996; 74: 318–323.

5. Kahan BD. Drug therapy: cyclosporine. N. Engl. J. Med. 1989; 321: 1725–1738.
6. Cho WY, Terasaki PI, Graver B. Fifteen-year kidney graft survival. In: Terasaki PI (ed.) Clinical Transplants. Los Angeles: UCLA Tissue Typing Laboratory: 1989; 325–331.
7. Myers BD, Newton L. Cyclosporine-induced chronic nephropathy: an obliterative microvascular injury. J. Am. Soc. Nephrol. 1991; 2(2 Suppl 1): S45–S52.
8. European FK506 Multicentre Liver Study Group. Randomised trial comparing tacrolimus (FK506) and cyclosporin in prevention of liver allograft rejection. Lancet. 1994; 344: 423–428.
9. The US Multicenter Liver FK506 Liver Study Group. A comparison of tacrolimus (FK506) and cyclosporine for immunosuppression in liver transplantation. N. Engl. J. Med. 1994; 331: 1110–1115.
10. Porayko MK, Texton SC, Krom RA et al. Nephrotoxic effects of primary immunosuppression with FK-506 and cyclosporine regimens after liver transplantation. Mayo. Clin. Proc. 1994; 69: 105–111.
11. Holman MJ, Gonwa TA, Cooper B et al. FK506-associated thrombotic thrombocytopenic purpura. Transplantation. 1993; 55: 205–206.
12. Ruggenenti P, Perico N, Mosconi L et al. Calcium channel blockers protect transplant patients from cyclosporine-induced daily renal hypoperfusion. Kidney Int. 1993; 43: 706–711.
13. Hoppu K, Koskimies O, Holmberg C, Hirvisalo EL. Pharmacokinetically determined cyclosporin dosage in young children. Pediatr. Nephrol. 1991; 5: 1–4.
14. Tejani A, Sullivan EK. Higher maintenance cyclosporine dose decreases the risk of graft failure in North American children: a report of the North American Pediatric Renal Transplant Cooperative Study. J. Am. Soc. Nephrol. 1996; 7: 550–555.
15. Chrysostomou A, Walker RG, Russ GR et al. Diltiazem in renal allograft recipients receiving cyclosporine. Transplantation. 1993; 55: 300–304.
16. Mourad G, Ribstein J, Mimran A. Converting-enzyme inhibitor versus calcium antagonist in cyclosporine-treated renal transplants. Kidney Int. 1993; 43: 419–425.
17. Houde I, Noel R, Cotret PR et al. Prednisone-mycophenolate mofetil double therapy for cyclosporine A toxicity in kidney transplantation. Transplantation. 1998; Suppl 139: abstract 243.
18. Ducloux D, Fournier V, Bresson-Vautrin C et al. Mycophenolate mofetil in renal transplant recipients with cyclosporine-associated nephrotoxicity. Transplantation. 1998; 65: 1504–1506.
19. Sheil A. Cancer in dialysis and transplant patients. In: Morris P (ed.) Kidney Transplantation: Principles and Practice, 4th edn. Philadelphia: WB Saunders; 1994: 390–400.
20. Penn I. The problem of cancer in organ transplant recipients: an overview. Transplant. Sci. 1994; 4: 23–32.
21. Penn I. The changing patterns of posttransplant malignancies. Transplant. Proc. 1991; 23: 1101–1103.
22. Penn I. Cancers complicating organ transplantation. N. Engl. J. Med. 1990; 323: 1767–1769.
23. McEnery P, Stablein P, Arbus G, Tejani A. Renal transplantation in children. A report of the North American Pediatric Renal transplant Cooperative Study. N. Engl. J. Med. 1992; 326: 1727–1732.
24. Tejani A, Sullivan EK, Alexander S, Fine R, Harmon W, Lilienfeld D. Post-transplant deaths and factors that influence the mortality rate in North American children. Transplantation. 1994; 57: 547–553.
25. Mullen DL, Silberg SG, Penn I, Hammond WS. Squamous cell carcinoma of the skin and lip in renal homograft recipients. Cancer. 1976; 37: 729–734.
26. Dantal J, Hourmant M, Cantarovich D et al. Effect of long-term immunosuppression in kidney-graft recipients on cancer incidence: randomised comparison of two cyclosporin regimens. Lancet. 1998; 351: 623–628.
27. Ho M, Jaffe R, Miller G et al. The frequency of Epstein-Barr virus infection and associated lymphoproliferative syndrome after transplantation and its manifestation in children. Transplantation. 1988; 45: 719–724.
28. Opelz G, Henderson R, for the Collaborative Transplant Study. Incidence of non-Hodgkin lymphoma in kidney and heart transplant recipients. Lancet. 1993; 342: 1514–1516.

29. Conlon PJ, Smith SR. Transmission of cancer with cadaveric donor organs. J. Am. Soc. Nephrol. 1995; 6: 54–60.
30. Gupta AK, Cardella CJ, Haberman HF. Cutaneous malignant neoplasms in patients with renal transplants. Arch. Dermatol. 1986; 122: 1288–1293.
31. Halmos O, Inturri P, Galligioni A et al. Two cases of Kaposi's sarcoma in renal and live transplant recipients treated with interferon. Clin. Transplant. 1996; 10: 374–378.
32. Tönshoff B, Mehls O. Interactions between glucocorticoids and the growth hormone – insulin-like growth factor axis. Pediatr. Transplant. 1997; 1: 183–188.
33. Tönshoff B, Mehls O. Factors affecting growth and strategies for treatment in children after renal transplantation. Pediatr. Transplant. 1997; 1: 176–182.
34. Tejani AH, Fine RN, Alexander S et al. Factors predictive of sustained growth in children after renal transplantation. J. Pediatr. 1993; 122: 397–402.
35. Hokken-Koelega ACS, van Zaal AE, de Ridder MAJ et al. Growth after renal transplantation in prepubertal children: impact of various treatment modalities. Pediatr. Res. 1994; 3: 367–371.
36. Broyer M, Guest G, Gagnadoux M-F. Growth rate in children receiving alternate-day cortico steroid treatment after kidney transplantation. J. Pediatr. 1992; 120: 721–725.
37. Jabs K, Sullivan EK, Avner ED, Harmon WE. Alternate-day steroid dosing improves growth without adversely affecting graft survival or long-term graft function. Transplantation. 1996; 61: 31–36.
38. Klare B, Strom TM, Hahn H et al. Remarkable long-term prognosis and excellent growth in kidney-transplant children under cyclosporine monotherapy. Transplant. Proc. 1991; 23: 1013–1017.
39. Ingulli E, Tejani AH. Steroid withdrawal after renal transplantation. In: Tejani AH, Fine RN (eds). Pediatric Renal Transplantation. New York: Wiley Liss, 1994; 221–238.
40. Shapiro R, Scantlebury VP, Jordan ML et al. FK 506 in pediatric kidney transplantation-Primary and rescue experience. Pediatr. Nephrol. 1995; 9: 43–48.
41. Grinyo JM, Gil-Vernet S, Seron D et al. Steroid withdrawal in mycophenolate mofetil-treated renal allograft recipients. Transplantation. 1997; 63: 1688–1690.
42. Tönshoff B, Mehls O. Use of rhGH post transplant in children. In: Tejani AH, Fine RN (eds). Pediatric Renal Transplantation. New York: Wiley & Sons, 1994; 441–460.
43. Tönshoff B, Haffner D, Mehls O et al. Efficacy and safety of growth hormone treatment in short children with renal allografts: three year experience. Kidney. Int. 1993; 44: 199–207.
44. Guest G, Berard E, Crosnier H, Chevallier T, Rappaport R, Broyer M. Effects of growth hormone in short children after renal transplantation. French Society of Pediatric Nephrology. Pediatr. Nephrol. 1998; 12: 437–446.
45. Tönshoff B. Editorial: The current status of mycophenolate mofetil in pediatric renal transplantation. Pediatr. Transplant. 1999, in press.

PART FIVE

Strategies

15.   Induction therapy

D. ABRAMOWICZ and K. M. WISSING

Induction therapy refers to the blocking of molecules involved in transplant immunity by an antibody or a soluble receptor during the peritransplant period. The critical biological event that characterizes the immediate post-transplant period is the increased expression of adhesion and co-stimulatory molecules, such as selectins, ICAMs, VCAMs and B7, throughout the graft as a consequence of the ischemia/reperfusion injury [1]. This may have two deleterious consequences. First, adhesion molecules are able to recruit and activate polymorphonuclear cells, a process which contributes to the development of delayed graft function. Second, the inflamed allograft may also promote the early migration and activation of alloreactive T cells, which may trigger acute rejection. Within this context, the possible actions of monoclonal antibodies or soluble receptor molecules that at present can not be matched by oral immunosuppressive drugs are:

(1) to maximally inhibit T cells during the initial weeks after transplantation, when the graft is most immunogenic;
(2) to target the adhesion molecules involved in the pathogenesis of delayed graft function;
(3) to help to achieve transplantation tolerance through the blockade of T-cell co-stimulation.

With regard to T cell blockade, there have been eight randomized, controlled trials of OKT3/ATG induction in renal transplantation performed to date [2–9]. While the majority showed a beneficial effect of induction on graft survival, only one [9] reached statistical significance, mainly because the other studies were of low statistical power. A meta-analysis of seven of the eight studies [10] has recently revealed a statistically significant and medically important 6% improvement of graft survival at 2 years after OKT3/ATG induction therapy, a figure yet to be achieved by any of the new immunosuppressive agents.

In fact, the benefits derived from OKT3/ATG induction are even higher under certain protocol conditions and in selected groups of patients. The first condition is that induction therapy has to be administered for a minimum period of time to lead to improved graft survival. Indeed, patients reported to the UNOS registry had a 5% increase of renal graft survival at 1 year only if OKT3/ATG therapy lasted for at least 5–7 days. Shorter periods did not result in improved graft survival [11]. Second, CsA must not be given together with

P. Cochat et al. (eds.), Immunosuppression under Trial, 125–129
©1999 Kluwer Academic Publishers.

OKT3 on the day of transplantation: the 5–15% increase of graft survival seen after OKT3 induction in the Collaborative Transplant Study registry was observed only if the introduction of CsA was delayed for some days after transplantation [12]. Whether this observation rests on an immunologic basis or is a consequence of the combined nephrotoxic effects of CsA and OKT3, and whether this deleterious interaction takes place with tacrolimus is still speculative. Of note, the same antagonism was also observed when polyclonal preparations were given on the same day as CsA [13]. Finally, OKT3/ATG induction has the greatest impact on graft survival in high immunological risk patients. When compared to the CsA–Sandimmune/azathioprine combination, OKT3 induction improved survival by 5% at 3 years in low-risk patients, defined as Caucasians, older than 15, not immunized, who received a first kidney with less than 36 h of cold ischemia time and no more than four HLA mismatches [13]. Much more striking improvements of long-term renal graft survival, reaching 15% and even more, were seen in high-risk patients such as blacks [12], children [12], immunized [9, 12], retransplanted [12, 14], those with two HLA-DR mismatches [6] or those receiving kidneys with long cold ischemia times [15]. These data were derived both from registries [12, 14] as well as from prospective, randomized trials [6, 9, 15]. With regard to the respective merits of OKT3 versus the polyclonal anti-lymphocyte preparations, data from the Collaborative Transplant Study registry suggest that OKT3 might be superior [13]. However, this could be related to the fact that some polyclonal anti-lymphocyte preparations are more potent than others as recently demonstrated in a double-blind comparison between rabbit thymoglobulin (IMTIX) and horse ATGAM (Upjohn) [16].

Whatever impressive these results may be, they were obtained in the CsA-Sandimmune/azathioprine era. Are there indications that the benefits are still present when induction therapy is given together with CsA-Neoral, tacrolimus, or MMF? Preliminary answers regarding rejection rates seem to be yes. The 20–25% incidence of rejection during the initial 6 months in patients receiving Neoral, MMF and steroids has been reduced to 11–14% with the addition of OKT3/ATG induction [17, 18]. Along the same lines, the 32% rejection rate observed with the tacrolimus/azathioprine/steroid combination was reduced to 18% in patients receiving ATG induction [19]. Thus, although we need to know more about the safety profile of these potent combinations, and whether they benefit some groups of patients more than others, it is already clear that OKT3/ATG induction will remain beneficial in the present era. With regard to the future, it will be important to evaluate the efficacy of variants of OKT3 which are non-immunogenic and non-activating, thereby not leading to the cytokine release syndrome. One such anti-CD3 mAb is undergoing a phase I trial [20].

More recently, several large trials have been performed with anti-interleukin-2 receptor (IL2R) mAbs as induction therapy in renal transplantation [21–23]. There are currently two such mAbs available: basiliximab (Simulect, Novartis), a chimeric IgG1 mAb, and daclizumab (Zenapax, Roche), which is a humanized IgG1 mAb. Both antibodies target the α chain of the trimeric IL2R complex, present only on activated T cells. Therefore, in opposition with OKT3/ATG Abs, anti-IL2R Abs should block only activated T cells, such as those engaged in the alloreactive response. Administration of only a few doses of these anti-IL2R mAbs were able to provide for up to 2 months of effective IL2R blockade. This long-term half life results from the absence of sensitization to these humanized or chimeric mAbs. A similar 35% reduction in the renal rejection rates at 6 months was observed with both antibodies in patients receiving CsA-Neoral as primary immunosuppression [21–23]. It must be noted, however, that 20% of the patients experienced rejection during the period of effective IL2R blockade with either antibody [23, 24]. Other pathways of T cell activation, possibly mediated by IL-15 and its receptor on T cells, might therefore be operative in this setting. Nevertheless, at present, anti-IL2R mAb therapy appears as effective as 6 months of continuous mycophenolate mofetil therapy for patients on CsA-Neoral. Future trials will tell how the anti-IL2R Abs compare with OKT3/ATG in high-risk patients, and whether they permit in combination with mycophenolate mofetil and steroids, the sparing of CsA or tacrolimus during the early post-transplant period.

Besides T cells, biological agents have also been used to target the adhesion/co-stimulatory molecules that trigger leucocyte migration within the inflamed post-ischemic graft where they may initiate delayed graft function. Several experimental data have shown that anti-ICAM-1 antibodies prevent neutrophil infiltration as well as post-ischemic renal failure in the rat. Anti-LFA-1 mAbs acted synergistically to prevent renal failure [25]. Interestingly, one clinical study in renal transplantation suggests that anti-LFA-1 mAbs might reduce the incidence of delayed graft function [26]. This trial compared a 10-day induction therapy with either ATG or a murine IgG1 anti-LFA-1 mAb. Anti-LFA-1 did not appear to be very immunosuppressive, as 11% of patients experienced rejection during its administration versus none in the ATG group. However, the incidence of delayed graft function was reduced from 35% in the ATG group to 19% in the anti-LFA-1 group. This prompted the IMTIX company to launch a prospective, randomized, double-blind, placebo-controlled study investigating the effect of the anti-LFA-1 mAb on the incidence of delayed graft function in patients at risk for this complication: specifically, those receiving grafts with more than 24 h of cold ischemia or from donors older than 50. If results are positive, this approach will be a significant breakthrough in solid organ transplantation.

Finally, one may expect that in the next decade, biological agents will help to induce transplantation tolerance. We know that T cells require a first signal delivered by the T cell receptor as well as second signals, provided by interactions between several possible costimulatory molecules, in order to proliferate and undergo clonal expansion. T cell unresponsiveness often occurs when the second signal is missing [27, 28]. While initial experiments show that blocking anti-LFA-1 and anti-ICAM-1 results in tolerance to murine cardiac allografts [29], it is now clear that the simultaneous blockade of both CD28/B7 and CD40/CD40-ligand interactions seems to be the most promising strategy for tolerance induction [27]. Indeed, immunosuppressive regimens blocking these two pathways have already been successful in achieving long-term renal allograft function in primates [30]. Phase I trials with molecules blocking the CD28/B7 and CD40/CD40-ligand pathways are ongoing in patients with autoimmune diseases [27], and one can hope that they will become a clinical reality in organ transplantation.

References

1. Fuggle SV, Koo DD. Cell adhesion molecules in clinical renal transplantation. Transplantation. 1998; 65: 763–769.
2. Michael J, Francos GC, Burke JF et al. A comparison of the effects of cyclosporine versus antilymphocyte globulin on delayed graft function in cadaver renal transplant recipients. Transplantation. 1989; 46: 805–808.
3. Belitsky AS, MacDonald AS, Cohen AD et al. Comparison of antilymphocyte globulin and continuous i.v. cyclosporin as induction immunosuppression for cadaver kidney transplants: a prospective randomized study. Transplant. Proc. 1991; 23: 999–1000.
4. Banhegyi C, Rockenschaub S, Muhlbacher F et al. Preliminary results of a prospective randomized clinical trial comparing cyclosporin A to antithymocyte globulin immunosuppressive induction therapy in kidney transplantation. Transplant. Proc. 1991; 23: 2207–2208.
5. Abramowicz D, Goldman M, De Pauw L, Vanherweghem J.L, Kinnaert P, Vereerstraeten P. The long-term effects of prophylactic OKT3 monoclonal antibody in cadaver kidney transplantation: A single-center, prospective, randomized study. Transplantation. 1992; 54: 433–437.
6. Norman DJ, Kahana L, Stuart FP et al. A randomized clinical trial of induction therapy with OKT3 in kidney transplantation. Transplantation. 1993; 55: 44–50.
7. Slakey DP, Johnson CP, Callaluce RD et al. A prospective randomized comparison of quadruple versus triple therapy for first cadaver transplants with immediate function. Transplantation. 1993; 56: 827–831.
8. Spanish Monotherapy Study Group. Cyclosporine monotherapy versus OKT3 and cyclosporine as induction therapy in older renal transplant patients: A multicenter randomized study. Transplant. Proc. 1994; 26: 2522–2524.
9. Thibaudin D, Alamartine E, de Filippis JP, Diab N, Blandine L, Berthoux F. Advantage of antithymocyte globulin induction in sensitized kidney recipients: a randomized prospective study comparing induction with and without antithymocyte globulin. Nephrol. Dial. Transplant. 1998; 13: 711–715.
10. Szczech LA, Berlin JA, Aradhye S, Grossmann RA, Feldman HI. Effect of anti-lymphocyte induction therapy on renal allograft survival: a meta-analysis. J. Am. Soc. Nephrol. 1997; 8: 1771–1777.
11. Shield CF, Edwards EB, Davies DB, Daily OP. Antilymphocyte induction therapy in cadaver renal transplantation. Transplantation. 1997; 63: 1257–1263.
12. Opelz G. Efficacy of rejection prophylaxis with OKT3 in renal transplantation. Transplantation. 1995; 60: 1220–1224.
13. Opelz G. Efficacy of rejection prophylaxis with OKT3 (letter). Transplantation. 1996; 62: 70.
14. Cecka JM, Gjertson D, Terasaki PI. Do prophylactic antilymphocyte globulins (ALG and OKT3) improve renal transplant survival in recipient and donor high-risk groups? Transplant. Proc. 1993; 25: 548–549.

15. Abramowicz D, Norman DJ, Vereerstraeten P et al. OKT3 prophylaxis in renal grafts with prolonged cold ischemia times: association with improvement in long-term survival. Kidney Int. 1996; 49: 768–772.
16. Gaber AO, First MR, Testi RJ, Gaston RS, Mendez R. Results of the double-blind randomized, multicenter, phase III clinical trial of thymoglobulin versus ATGAM in the treatment of acute graft rejection episodes after renal transplantation. Transplantation. 1998; 66: 29–37.
17. Lebranchu Y et al. A randomized, double-blind, multicenter trial comparing two corticosteroid regimens in combination with mycophenolate mofetil (MMF) and cyclosporine (CYA) in renal transplant recipients. Transplantation Society XVII congress 1998; abstract book p. 14.
18. Henry ML, Elkhammas EA, Bumgardner GL, Davies EA, Pelletier RP, Ferguson RM. Antibody induction in the current era. Transplantation. 1998; 65: S65.
19. Charpentier B et al. A randomized multicenter trial of Tacrolimus in renal transplantation comparing induction vs. non-induction therapy. Transplantation Society XVII congress 1998; Abstract book p. 115.
20. Pescovitz MD et al. Safety of the new antibodies. Transplantation Society XVII congress 1998; Abstract book p. 90.
21. Nashan B, More R, Amlot P, Schmidt AG, Abeywickrama K, Soulillou JP. Randomised trial of basiliximab versus placebo for control of acute cellular rejection in renal allograft recipients. Lancet. 1997; 350: 1193–1198.
22. Vincenti F, Kirkman R, Light S et al. Interleukin-2-receptor blockade with daclizumab to prevent acute rejection in renal transplantation. N. Engl. J. Med. 1998; 338: 161–165.
23. Nashan B, Light S, Hardie IR, Lin A, Johnson JR. Reduction of acute renal allograft rejection by daclizumab. Transplantation. 1999; 67: 110–115.
24. Kovarik JM, Gerbeau C, Hall M, Schmidt AG. Influence of the duration of IL-2 receptor (IL-2R) blockade on the incidence of acute rejection episodes in renal transplantation. Transplantation. 1998; 65: S179.
25. Kelly KJ, Williams WW, Colvin RB, Bonventre JV. Antibody to intercellular adhesion molecule 1 protects the kidney against ischemic injury. Proc. Natl. Acad. Sci. USA. 1994; 91: 812–816.
26. Hourmant M, Bedrossian J, Durand D et al. A randomized multicenter trial comparing leucocyte function-associated antigen-1 monoclonal antibody with rabbit antithymocyte globulin as induction treatment in first kidney transplantations. Transplantation. 1996; 62: 1565–1570.
27. Sayegh MH, Turka LA. The role of T-cell costimulatory activation pathways in transplant rejection. N. Engl. J. Med. 1998; 1813–1821.
28. Alegre ML. Costimulatory molecules as targets for the induction of transplantation tolerance. Nephrol. Dial. Transplant. 1999; 14: 322–332.
29. Isobe M, Yagita H, Okumura K, Ihara A. Specific acceptance of cardiac allograft after treatment with antibodies to ICAM-1 and LFA-1. Science. 1992; 255: 1125–1127.
30. Kirk AD, Harlan DM, Amstrong NN. CTLA4-Ig and anti-CD40 ligand prevent renal allograft rejection in primates. Proc. Natl. Acad. Sci. USA. 1997; 94: 8789–8794.

16. Effect of long-term immunosuppression in kidney-graft recipients on cancer incidence: randomised comparison of two cyclosporin regimens*

J. DANTAL, M. HOURMANT, D. CANTAROVICH, M. GIRAL,
G. BLANCHO, B. DRENO and J.-P. SOULILLOU

Introduction

The introduction of cyclosporin into maintenance therapy for kidney-transplant recipients has played an important part in the improvement of graft survival reported worldwide [1]. Cyclosporin is potentially toxic to various tissues including kidney, liver, endocrine pancreas, and nervous system, and its use is associated with hypertension [2]. Nevertheless, the capacity of cyclosporin treatment to increase graft survival has been recognised for a long time. Optimum doses and trough blood concentrations of cyclosporin have been empirically evolved so as to cause the least kidney toxicity. However, cyclosporin has other potential side-effects related to its immunosuppressant properties, including the occurrence of infections and tumours. The magnitude of these effects may also vary with dose and consequent trough blood concentrations. Thus, there is potential for improvement in dose schedules. In terms of reducing long-term complications of immunosuppression, such as cancers [3], kidney recipients are unlike other organ-graft recipients because long-term dialysis is a viable alternative.

The aim of this prospective, open, randomised study was to assess the benefits and risks of two maintenance (ie, 1 year after transplantation) treatment strategies: in the normal-dose group cyclosporin doses yield trough concentrations within the generally recommended range (150–250 ng/mL) and in the low-dose group the trough blood concentrations were half those of the normal-dose group (ie, 75–125 ng/mL).

Patients and methods

Patients

Between December, 1989 and December, 1994, we considered for inclusion patients who underwent first-time kidney transplantation, were older than 18

*This paper was first published in *The Lancet* 1998; 357: 623–28 (February 28), and is reprinted here by kind permission. © by The Lancet Ltd. 1998.

P. Cochat et al. (eds.), Immunosuppression under Trial, 131–144
©1999 Kluwer Academic Publishers.

years, and who gave informed consent. Reasons for exclusion were more than one acute rejection episode before enrolment, recurrence of the initial disease in the graft or proteinuria of more than 1 g/day, 1-year serum creatinine concentrations above 250 μmol/L, and neoplasia diagnosed during the first year after transplantation. We also excluded non-resident patients unavailable for regular follow-up in our centre, patients enrolled in other studies, and those unwilling to participate. The study was approved by our local ethics committee. Since our institution uses a two-drug regimen (principally cyclosporin and azathioprine without steroids) after the third month [4, 5], and because of the potential risk of acute or chronic rejection after the reduction of immunosuppression, the change in cyclosporin maintenance dose was randomly introduced 1 year after grafting, and was restricted to patients who had experienced no more than one episode of acute interstitial rejection during the year.

Protocol

Immediate post-transplantation treatment was with antithymocyte globulins (IMTIX, Lyon, France; 91%), monoclonal antibodies (7%) [6, 7], or cyclosporin starting from the first day (2%). Steroids, starting at 1 mg/kg daily, were tapered and stopped around day 90. At 1 year, the patients were receiving either cyclosporin plus azathioprine (77%), cyclosporin plus prednisolone (if intolerant of azathioprine; 18%), or cyclosporin alone (5%). The principal investigators held a set of sealed envelopes containing the randomisation code. The envelopes were opened after informed consent was obtained. Only two patients refused to join the study. Both investigators and participating patients were aware of treatment allocation. Randomisation was carried out with stratification for age ($\leq$ 50 or > 50 years), panel-reactive antibodies ($\leq$ 75% or > 75%), serum creatinine ($\leq$ 150 μmol/L or > 150 μmol/L), and presence or absence of an acute interstitial rejection episode in the first year after transplantation.

Doses of cyclosporin were administered so as to yield trough concentrations of 75–125 ng/mL for the low-dose group and 150–250 ng/mL for the normal-dose group. Cyclosporin in its native form was monitored by measurement of whole-blood concentrations (Cyclo-Trac SP Whole Blood, Incstar, Stillwater, USA) measured 12 h after the last oral dose (trough concentrations). In addition, 6 h areas under curve (AUC) of blood cyclosporin concentrations were calculated at inclusion and every 6 months, by means of Siphar-win (version 1.13) software. The equivalence of the two groups in terms of azathioprine doses was also monitored by AUC of blood 6-mercaptopurine concentration (the major azathioprine metabolite), white-blood-cell count, and mean corpuscular volume.

When acute rejection episodes occurred, first-line therapy was steroid boluses [8]. Rescue therapy in steroid-resistant episodes was with antithymocyte globulin, 1.25 mg/kg daily for 10 days.

Follow-up

All patients were clinically examined at inclusion and every 6 months thereafter; particular attention was paid to skin lesions. All female patients underwent gynaecological examination and mammography at the end of follow-up. Trough blood cyclosporin concentrations were monitored twice a month during the first 3 months after enrolment and reduction of cyclosporin doses and then every 2 months. The mean duration of follow-up after transplantation was 66 (SD 18) months for both groups (range 36–96; median 68).

Renal function and rejection

Renal function was analysed every 6 months by comparison of serum creatinine concentrations, Cockroft calculated creatinine clearance, and the reciprocal serum creatinine ratio. Although graft histology was available in each case of rejection, the definition of acute rejection was the introduction of antirejection therapy. Chronic rejection was defined as chronic renal dysfunction – after exclusion of all other causes of renal damage – as identified by a slow decrease in renal function unresponsive to the maximum reduction of cyclosporin doses permitted within the range of the relevant experimental protocol.

Statistical methods

The primary endpoint was graft function. Secondary endpoints were survival of patients, graft survival, frequency of malignant disorders, and frequency of infection episodes. The analysis was done after the last patient completed 3 years of follow-up.

The sample size was estimated with the assumption that the mean serum creatinine in the low-dose group would be 15% below that in the normal-dose group at 2–3 years. The type-1 error rate (α) was taken to be 0.05 and the power required was 80%. Under these conditions, the number of patients required was 100. The baseline data in the two groups of patients were compared by means of Student's t test for continuous data and the χ^2 for categorical variables. Differences in survival were assessed (not censored for deaths) for statistical significance by Kaplan-Meier survival analysis (log-rank test), which was also used to compare the profiles of onset of neoplasia after transplantation. We used the Cox semi-parametric model to study the influence of prognostic factors on the appearance of neoplasia and the Cochrane-Mantel-Haenszel test to compare the frequency of neoplasia in the two groups (with adjustment for the azathioprine dose). To avoid possible bias, renal-function data (including patients with graft loss) were adjusted for the predialysis serum creatinine value [9]. For the creatinine clearance study, patients were classified as score 0 for values below 25 mL/min, 1 for values of 25–50 mL/min, 2 for values above 50 mL/min, and 3 for dialysis. The Wilcoxon non-parametric test was used to compare the score distribution in the two groups.

Results

Of 425 consecutive transplant recipients, 194 did not meet the inclusion criteria. 231 patients were enrolled and randomly assigned normal-dose or low-dose cyclosporin (Figure 1).

In the absence of the precise knowledge of the overall effect of our protocol, some events that occurred after the study started were considered as grounds to change treatment. Patients with acute rejection (ten), clinical recurrence of initial disease (four), cancer (except for patients with skin cancer and fewer than three lesions; 17 patients), or pregnancy (five) during the study had their treatment adjusted, for instance, by a change to the normal-dose regimen for acute rejection, or withdrawal of immunosuppressants in post-transplant lympho-proliferative disorders. However, these patients were not withdrawn from the study and their outcome is given in the analysis (intention-to-treat study).

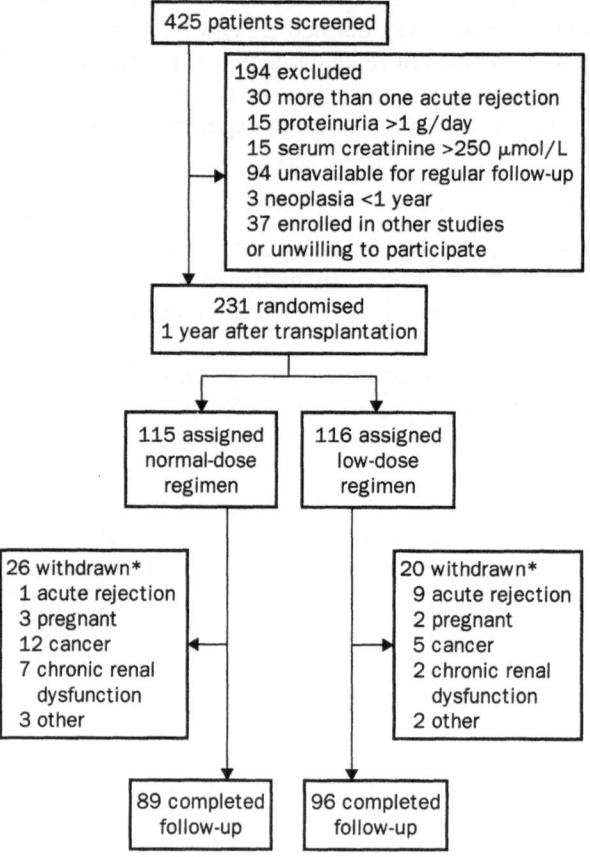

Fig. 1.   Trial profile. *Included in analysis despite withdrawal from treatment

The two randomised groups were similar in terms of pretransplantation clinical and immunological variables except the duration of dialysis (Table 1). The duration was longer in the normal-dose than in the low-dose group, mainly because more patients in that group had been on long-term dialysis (more than 10 years; nine *vs* one). 46 patients in the normal-dose group and 50 in the low-dose group had been on dialysis for less than a year. The two groups did not differ in their initial disease distribution, notably for glomerulonephritis treated before transplantation with immunosuppressant and cytotoxic drugs – regimens that could have resulted in delayed malignant disorders. Eight patients in the normal-dose group and 13 in the low-dose group had glomerulonephritis; three and six, respectively, had received steroids; five in each group had received cyclophosphamide or chlorambucil; and two in the low-dose group had received cyclosporin. The two groups were also similar in terms of donor and graft characteristics, clinical outcome in the recipient during the first year after transplantation, and graft function at the time of inclusion (Table 1).

Monitoring of immunosuppressive regimen

At trial entry, the normal-dose and low-dose groups did not differ in mean cyclosporin dose (5.2 [SD 1.8] *vs* 4.9 [1.7] mg/kg daily), trough concentration (199 [57] *vs* 202 [53] ng/mL), or AUC (3166 [1016] *vs* 3017 [814] h ng mL^{-1}). The desired ranges of cyclosporin trough concentrations were obtained within 3 months of trial entry and remained stable thereafter (Figure 2); there was only 8.5% overlap between the groups after 6 months. The mean cyclosporin AUC was higher in the normal-dose group than the low-dose group at 6 months (3234 [1142] *vs* 2028 [709] h ng mL^{-1}) and throughout follow-up. In the low-dose group, the 51.7% (12.8) decrease in trough cyclosporin concentration was obtained with a reduction of only 27.2% (16.0) in dose. The number of patients receiving both cyclosporin and azathioprine did not change during follow-up in either group, but doses of azathioprine decreased slightly from 1.2 (0.5) mg/kg daily in both groups at trial entry to 1.09 (0.5) mg/kg daily in the low-dose group and 1.02 (0.5) mg/kg daily in the normal-dose group at 6 years. Furthermore, there were no differences between the groups in AUC of 6-mercaptopurine, white-blood-cell count, or mean corpuscular volume; these findings confirm the equivalence of azathioprine exposure in the two groups.

Graft function

There was no significant differences between the groups in the evolution of renal function, in terms of mean serum creatinine, ratio, or linear regression. However, there was a significant differences in creatinine clearance between 6 and 42 months ($p > 0.03$, data not shown), which suggests that some cyclosporin nephrotoxicity occurred in patients on the normal-dose regimen. At 66 months of follow-up mean serum creatinine (182 [SD 160] *vs* 184 [157] μmol/L,

Table 1.   Pretransplantation clinical and immunological variables

Variable	Normal-dose group (n = 115)	Low-dose group (n = 116)
Demography		
Mean (range) age (years)	47.8 (20–69)	47.9 (18–69)
Male/female	62/53	66/50
Mean (range) time on dialysis (months)	31.5 (0–204)	21.5 (0–120)
Donor and transplant characteristics		
Mean (SD) donor age (years)	34.1 (12.8)	35.7 (14.3)
Mean (SD) HLA incompatibility index		
A	1.05 (0.66)	1.04 (0.62)
B	1.29 (0.67)	1.39 (0.68)
DR	0.97 (0.66)	1.00 (0.66)
Patients with historical, positive, cross match	6	3
Mean (SD) cold ischaemia time (h)	33.7 (10.1)	34.4 (9.7)
Induction treatment		
Antithymocyte globulin*	102	108
Anti-CD4	5	3
Anti-LFA1	5	1
Cyclosporin on day 0	3	1
Mean (SD) day cyclosporin introduced	9.3 (4.0)	9.3 (5.0)
Mean (SD) delay in graft function (days)	6.0 (6.1)	5.7 (6.2)
Rejection episodes before trial entry		
Number of recipients with rejection†	23 (20%)	24 (20.7%)
Mean (SD) day on onset of rejection episode	60 (42)	68 (71)
Mean (SD) day of cyclosporin withdrawal	92 (65)	91 (63)
Viral infections before trial entry		
Cytomegalovirus	28 (24.3%)	24 (20.7%)
Human herpesvirus 1 and 2	34 (29.6%)	29 (25.0%)
Mean (SD) azathioprine dose at inclusion (mg/kg)	1.2 (0.49)	1.2 (0.47)
Kidney function		
Mean (SD) serum creatinine at inclusion (μmol/L)	133 (38)	140 (39)
< 150 μmol/L	81	78
150–200 μmol/L	25	29
> 200 μmol/L	9	10

Data are number of patients otherwise stated.
*Mean duration 10.9 days (SD 4.0) in both groups.
†All episodes treated with cyclosporin boluses; two patients received additional antithymocyte globulin therapy; no CKT3 rescue

p = 0.9) and creatinine clearance (47.5 [25.1] *vs* 45.3 [22.5] mL/min; p = 0.6) were similar in the low-dose and normal-dose groups. By contrast, more patients in the low-dose group than in the normal-dose group were treated for acute rejection episodes (nine *vs* one, p < 0.02), although there was no detrimental influence on actuarial graft survival (89 *vs* 82% at 6 years). Acute rejection was defined as any episode that necessitated the introduction of antirejection therapy; however, retrospective histological analysis confirmed the presence of acute rejection in seven of the nine treated episodes (78%) in the low-dose group,

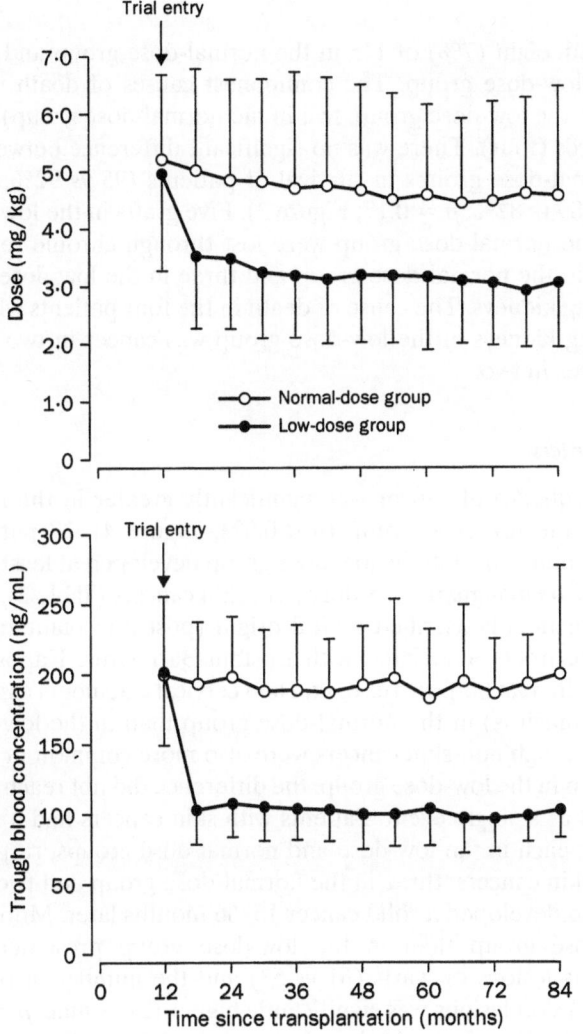

Fig. 2. Cyclosporin dose and trough blood concentrations. Bar = SD

one being borderline and the six grade I according to the Banff classification [10]. The two other patients had a histological pattern of chronic rejection and had therefore been incorrectly treated for acute rejection. Chronic renal dysfunction was diagnosed in 11 patients in the low-dose group (four grafts still functioning) and in 15 patients in the normal-dose group (six still functioning). Recurrence of initial glomerulonephritis (confirmed by biopsy) occurred in 12 normal-dose and nine low-dose patients.

Survival

15 patients died, eight (7%) of 115 in the normal-dose group and seven (6%) of 116 in the low-dose group. The commonest causes of death were cancer (seven – two in the low-dose group, five in the normal-dose group) and cardio-vascular diseases (four). There was no significant difference between the low-dose and normal-dose groups in survival of patients (95 *vs* 92%; $p = 0.7$) or graft survival (89 *vs* 82%; $p = 0.17$; Figure 3). Five grafts in the low-dose group and eight in the normal-dose group were lost through chronic rejection, and eight patients in the normal-dose group and three in the low-dose group died with functioning kidneys. The cause of death in the four patients who died with non-functioning kidneys in the low-dose group was cancer in two and cardio-vascular diseases in two.

Malignant disorders

The overall frequency of cancer was significantly greater in the normal-dose group than in the low-dose group ($p < 0.034$, Figure 4). 37 patients in the normal-dose group and 23 in the low-dose group developed at least one cancer. 43 (66%) of the 65 malignant disorders were skin cancers (Table 2). There were more cancers generally ascribed a viral origin (post-transplantation lympho-proliferative disorders associated with Epstein-Barr virus, Kaposi's sarcoma associated with human herpesvirus 8, skin and cervical carcinoma associated with human papillomavirus) in the normal-dose group than in the low-dose group ($p = 0.05$). Although non-skin cancers were also more common in the normal-dose group than in the low-dose group, the difference did not reach significance when analysed as a single event. Patients with skin cancers had a mean of 1.9 and 2.1 lesions each in the low-dose and normal-dose groups, respectively. Of patients with skin cancers, three in the normal-dose group and two in the low-dose group also developed a solid cancer 15–66 months later. More patients in the normal-dose group than in the low-dose group presented with pre-epitheliomatous lesions or warts (61 *vs* 53) and the number of patients with multiple (> 10) skin lesions was significantly higher (21 *vs* nine, $p < 0.02$). Two patients who withdrew from the low-dose group at 3 months and 14 months because of rejection episodes (treated with steroid boluses) developed, res-pectively, a post-transplantation lymphoproliferative disorder and a Merckel-cell tumour (cutaneous neuroendocrine carcinoma), 49 and 55 months after inclusion. These patients were subsequently changed to the normal-dose cyclosporin regimen but their data are included in the low-dose group. Cancer was more frequent in recipients older than 50 years than in younger patients ($p < 0.0001$), in men than in women ($p < 0.004$), and in patients who received the highest mean doses of azathioprine ($p < 0.03$). No other recipient or donor characteristics (Table 1) studied were found to be significant. The Cox semi-parametric model confirmed that the normal-dose group was at a higher risk of cancer than the low-dose group ($p < 0.026$).

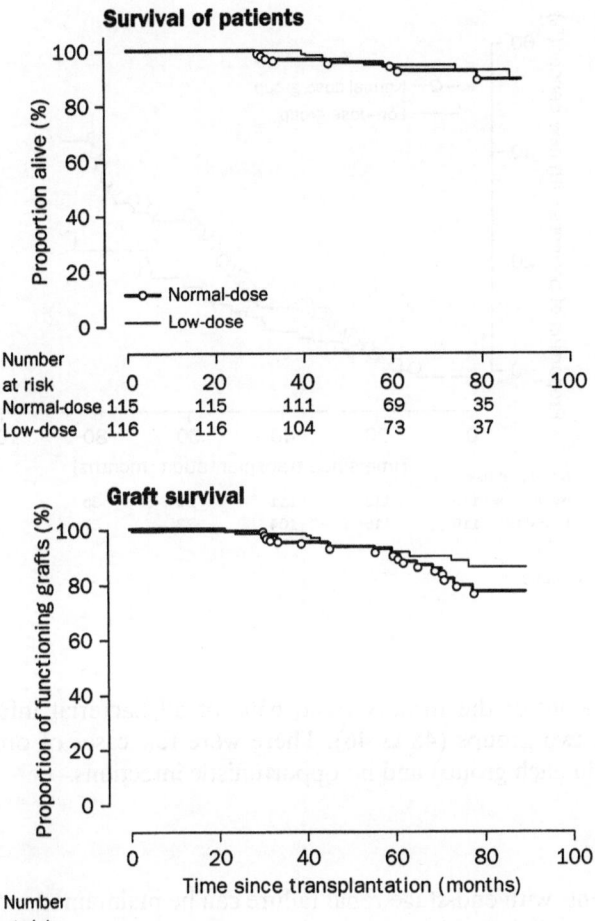

Fig. 3. Survival of patients and graft survival

Laboratory findings and infections

Blood pressure and the need for antihypertensive treatment were not significantly affected by the cyclosporin regimen. Cholesterol and triglyceride concentrations were slightly but not significantly lower in the low-dose group than in the normal-dose group. Episodes of virus infection (human herpesviruses 1 and 2, herpes zoster) were more frequent in patients in the normal-dose group (16 *vs* nine, $p < 0.04$); no overt cytomegalovirus infection was diagnosed after trial entry. The number of patients who developed bacterial

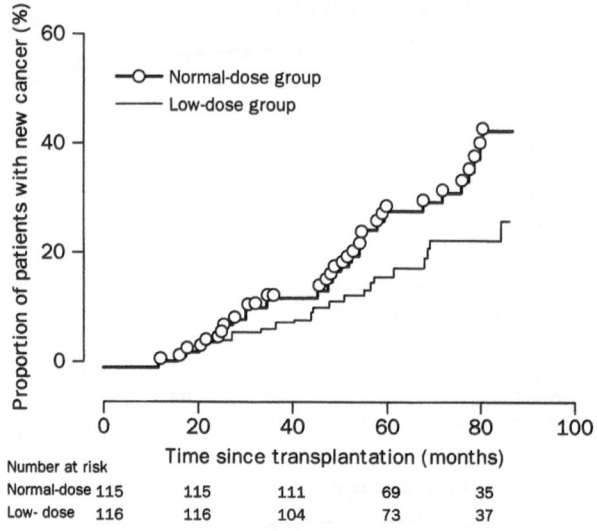

Fig. 4.   Frequency of cancer

Number at risk				
Normal-dose 115	115	111	69	35
Low- dose 116	116	104	73	37

infections (mainly of the urinary tract, 65% of all bacterial infections) was similar in the two groups (48 *vs* 46). There were few cases of oropharyngeal mycosis (two in each group) and no opportunistic infections.

Discussion

Because patients with end-stage renal failure can be maintained indefinitely on long-term haemodialysis, kidney-transplant recipients may have a very different view – compared with recipients of heart or liver transplants – about the acceptability of complications of excessive immunosuppression. Although some centres have used cyclosporin monotherapy [11] or a combination of cyclosporin and azathioprine once graft function is in steady state [12], the majority of centres use triple therapy (cyclosporine, azathioprine,and steroids) [13].

The association between immunosuppression in graft recipients and an increased risk of malignant disorders has long been known [13, 14]. As well as the part played by induction treatments with such powerful immunosuppressants as antithymocyte globulin and monoclonal antibodies to CD3 [15], maintenance treatment may also have an important role in these life-threatening late complications. A detailed reappraisal of the delayed risk of long-term immunosuppression in kidney-transplant recipients is also called for since the introduction of a new formulation of cyclosporin (Neoral), which increases bioavailability and exposure to the drug [16], the availability of new

Table 2. Distribution of cancers

Type of cancer	Number of patients	
	Normal-dose group (n = 115)	Low-dose group (n = 116)
Skin cancers		
Squamous-cell carcinoma	15	8
Bowen's disease	2	5
Basal-cell carcinoma	9	4
All skin cancers*	26	17
Cervical intraepithelial neoplasia	1	1
Kaposi's sarcoma	1	0
Post-transplantation lymphoproliferative disorder		
Mucosa-associated	1	0
Non-Hodgkin lymphoma	2	1†
All	3	1
Other cancers		
Breast	4	1
Adenocarcinoma of unknown origin	2	0
Uterus	0	1
Prostate	0	1
Oral	1	1
Kidney	1	0
Lung	0	1
Merckel-cell	1	1
Total	9	6
Total		
With at least one cancer	37	23
With more than one cancer type	3	2

*Total number of skin-cancer lesions 54 in normal-dose group, 32 in low-dose group.
†Transferred to normal-dose treatment after undergoing a rejection episode

drugs, and the use of combinations of these new drugs [17–19]. In addition, some investigators, less concerned about long-term cyclosporin nephrotoxicity, argue that cyclosporin doses should be maintained above a threshold of 4 mg/kg daily [9]. Although all drugs might not have exactly similar effects (eg, some could have antiproliferative effects [20–22]), the new regimens carry the potential threat of a parallel diminution in the immune surveillance of malignant cells in a biological environment that is also more permissive towards chronic oncogenic viral infections.

Our findings from this single-centre randomised prospective study may underestimate the actual risk of cancer. These patients had good graft outcome 1 year after transplantation and they did not receive the most aggressive immunosuppression during the first year (before randomisation) – we excluded patients who had had more than one rejection episode, and none had received triple therapy. There were no differences between the groups in doses of the associated azathioprine or steroids.

The frequency of acute cellular rejection was significantly higher in the low-dose group than in the normal-dose group. There was no clear predictive factor for the occurrence of such episodes after reduction of the cyclosporin dose (such as the occurrence of a first rejection in the prerandomisation first year, the level of pregraft panel-reactive antibodies, or the HLA matching). Although renal function in the two groups was similar at 6 years, we cannot rule out the possibility that these episodes of late acute rejection will affect long-term graft outcome [23]. Since the risk may have been underestimated as a result of the small numbers of patients and events, careful monitoring of patients receiving a low-dose regimen is necessary. This finding also retrospectively justified the restrictions we imposed on entry to the trial. We were surprised that the halving of trough blood cyclosporin concentrations resulted in only a slight and non-significant improvement in the usual indices of kidney-graft function (serum creatinine); only the comparison of creatinine clearance calculated by Cockroft's method showed a significant difference from the normal-dose group.

Our main finding was the significantly lower frequency of cancer in patients treated with the low-dose cyclosporin regimen. Since the survey time averaged only about 6.5 years, the final risk is probably underestimated. The frequency of cancers common in the general population was also lower in the low-dose group than in the normal-dose group but the difference did not reach significance. About two-thirds of the cancers observed were skin carcinomas. This proportion of skin cancers over all other de-novo neoplasms is higher than the rate of 50% reported in other series [14, 24, 25], perhaps because ill patients were specifically examined for skin lesions during our study. Although never life-threatening in our series, many of the skin carcinomas were recurrent; in five cases lesions appeared a few months before the development of a second, non-skin, cancer. Furthermore, the occurrence of carcinoma was not influenced by whether antirejection therapy was given before randomisation (including prophylactic treatment), the type of such therapy, or pretransplantation immuno-suppressive treatment of glomerulonephritis, although there were more cancers among patients who had received the highest doses of azathioprine, as suggested previously [26]. No patient died from skin cancer, but many of the other cancers were life-threatening with aggressive presentations (clinical or histological), and there were seven deaths. Our finding that cancer was the main cause of death is not inconsistent with the results of a previous survey in which vascular diseases were the commonest cause of death [27], since deaths before trial entry (1 year after transplantation) were not included in ours study.

An increased risk of de-novo neoplasia after transplantation has been reported previously [14]. The increased rate is a result mainly of virus-induced malignant disorders [28]. A possible explanation is that the high degree of immunosuppression results in diminished immune surveillance of virus-transformed cells, an increase in the frequency of virus infection or of viral load in transplant recipients, or both factors. However, the risk of other types of cancer (ie, not virus linked) is also increased [24, 29] with the exception of breast cancer [30]. The three main factors affecting the risk of de-novo neoplasia in transplant recipients, also found in or study, are the patient's age, sex, and length of exposure to immunosuppressant drugs after transplantation [25]. Age is important because the mean age of transplant patients has increased (8.3% patients older than 55 years before 1981 compared with 24.8% after 1994, in our centre). Long-term survival is also steadily improving, further increasing the length of exposure. Our prospective study has also shown that the frequency of cancer is also directly related to the degree of immuno-suppression, and suggests that the widely accepted range of trough cyclosporin concentrations may be too high.

The possibility that the reported effect is restricted to the use of cyclosporin seems highly unlikely. For example, the rate of post-transplantation lympho-proliferative disorders seems to be related to excessive immunosuppression; an increase occurs each time a new immunosuppressive agent is introduced, particularly during the 'learning' phase when high doses are used. The frequency of cancer might be expected to increase whenever new, powerful treatments – whether new compounds or new combinations – are introduced.

References

1. The Canadian Multicentre Transplant Study Group. A randomized clinical trial of cyclosporine in cadaveric renal transplantation. N. Engl. J. Med. 1986; 314: 1219–1225.
2. Bennett WM, De Mattos A, Meyer MM et al. Chronic cyclosporine nephropathy: the Achilles' heel of immunosuppressive therapy. Kidney Int. 1996; 50: 1089–1100.
3. Sheil AGR, Disney APS, Mathew TH et al. De novo malignancy emerges as a major cause of morbidity and late failure in renal transplantation. Transplant. Proc. 1993; 25: 1383–1384.
4. Hourmant M, Taupin JL, Lemergie D et al. Azathioprine-cyclosporine A (CyA) double therapy versus CyA alone after the first rejection episode in kidney-transplanted patients under CyA: a randomized study. Transplant. Int. 1989; 2: 113–116.
5. Opeiz G. Effect of the maintenance immunosuppressive drug regimen on kidney transplant outcome. Transplantation. 1994; 58: 443–446.
6. Hourmant M, Le Mauff B, Lemeur Y et al. Administration of an anti-CD11a monoclonal antibody in recipients of kidney transplantation: a pilot study. Transplantation. 1994: 58: 377–380.
7. Dantal J, Ninin E, Hourmant M et al. Anti-CD4 MoAb therapy in kidney transplantation: a pilot study in early prophylaxis of rejection. Transplantation. 1996; 62: 1502–1506.
8. Soulillou JP, Cantarovich D, Lemauff B et al. Randomized controlled trial of a monoclonal antibody against the interleukin-2 receptor (33B3.1) as compared with rabbit antithymocyte globulins for prophylaxis against rejection of renal allografts. N. Engl. J. Med. 1990; 322: 1175–1182.
9. Burcke JF, Pirsch JD, Ramos EL et al. A multicenter four year retrospective study in renal transplant recipients treated with cyclosporine. evidence for long term efficacy and safety. N. Engl. J. Med. 1994; 331: 358–363.
10. Solez K, Axelsen RA, Benediktsson H et al. International standardization of criteria for the histologic diagnosis of renal allograft rejection: the Banff working classification of kidney transplant pathology. Kidney Int. 1993; 44: 411–422.
11. European Multicenter Trial Group. Cyclosporin in cadaveric renal transplantation: 1 year follow-up of a multicentre trial. Lancet. 1983; ii: 986–989.
12. Kasiske BL, Heim-Duthoy KL, Ma JZ. Elective cyclosporine withdrawal after renal transplantation: a metaanalysis. JAMA. 1993; 269: 395–400.
13. Lindholm A, Ohlman S, Albrechtsen D et al. The impact of acute rejection episodes on long-

term graft function and outcome in 1347 primary renal transplants treated by 3 cyclosporine regimens. Transplantation. 1993; 56: 307–315.

14. Penn I. Occurrence of cancers in immunosuppressed organ transplant recipients In: Tearaski PI, Cecka JM eds. Clinical transplants. Los Angeles: UCLA Tissue Typing Laboratory, 1994; 99–109.

15. Opelz G, Henderson R. Incidence of non-Hodgkin lymphoma in kidney and heart transplant recipients. Lancet. 1993; 342: 1514–1516.

16. Kovarik JM, Mueller EA, Van Bree JB et al. Cyclosporine pharmacokinetics and variability from a microemulsion formulation: a multicenter investigation in kidney transplant patients. Transplantation. 1994; 58: 658–663.

17. The Tricontinental Mycophenolate Mofetil Renal Transplantation Study Group. A blinded, randomized clinical trial of mycophenolate mofetil for the prevention of acute rejection in cadaveric renal transplantation. Transplantation. 1996; 61: 1029–1037.

18. Vincenti F, Laskow DA, Neylan JF et al. One-year-follow-up of an open-label trial of FK 506 for primary kidney transplantation. Transplantation. 1996; 61: 1576–1581.

19. Kahan BD. Sirolimus: a new agent for clinical renal transplantation. Transplant. Proc. 1997; 29: 36–41.

20. Morris RE. Beware: shifting paradigms ahead. Lancet. 1996; 348 (suppl. II): II26.

21. Dilling MB, Dias P, Shapiro DN et al. Rapamycin selectively inhibits the growth of childhood rhabdomyosarcoma cells through inhibition of signaling via the insulin like growth factor receptor. Cancer Res. 1994; 54: 903–908.

22. Tressler RJ, Garvin LJ, Slate DL. Anti-tumor activity of mycophenolate mofetil against human and mouse tumors in vivo. Int. J. Cancer. 1994; 57: 568–573.

23. Cecka JM, Cho YW, Terasaki PI. Analyses of the UNOS scientific renal transplant registry at three years–early events affecting transplant success. Transplantation. 1992; 53: 59–64.

24. London NJ, Farmery SM, Will EJ et al. Risk of neoplasia in renal transplant patients. Lancet. 1995; 346: 403–406.

25. Blohme I, Larkö O. Premalignant and malignant skin lesions in renal transplant patients. Transplantation. 1984; 37: 165–167.

26. Confavreux C, Saddier P, Grimaud J et al. Risk of cancer from azathioprine therapy in multiple sclerosis: a case-control study. Neurology. 1996; 46: 1607–1612.

27. West M, Sutherland D, Matas A. Kidney transplant recipients who die with functioning grafts. Transplantation. 1996; 62: 1019–1030.

28. Morris JDH, Eddleston ALWF, Crook T. Viral infection and cancer. Lancet. 1995; 346: 754–758.

29. Buccianti G, Ravasi B, Cresseri D et al. Cancer in patients on renal replacement therapy in Lombardy, Italy. Lancet. 1996; 347: 59–60.

30. Stewart T, Tsai SCJ, Grayson H et al. Incidence of de-novo breast cancer in women chronically immunosuppressed after organ transplantation. Lancet. 1995; 346: 796–798.

17. Immunosuppression in composite tissue transplantation

J. M. DUBERNARD, E. R. OWEN, N. LEFRANÇOIS, P. PETRUZZO,
X. MARTIN, M. DAWAHRA, D. JULLIEN, J. KANITAKIS,
J.-M. RAMACKERS, X. PREVILLE, L. GEBUHRER, J.-F. NICOLAS,
N. HAKIM and J.-P. REVILLARD

Introduction

Composite tissue allografts (CTA) are defined as neurovascularized allografts of non vital tissues which include structural, functional and aesthetic units of integumentary and musculoskeletal elements, e.g. hand or larynx [1].

Limb transplantation, the most common experimental model of CTA, has met with variable different degrees of success. Advances in microsurgical techniques suggest that the technical problems can be favorably overcome, as demonstrated by successful hand reimplantation in man (autografts) [2].

The potential human applications for CTA are numerous in functional and anatomical reconstruction of many peripheral tissue defects following traumatic injuries, major burns, cancers or birth abnormalities.

The immunological issues of the CTA are extremely complex as different tissues are involved, each of which has to be considered individually as well as part of an unity presenting different time and strength of rejection [1]. Cartilage, ligaments and fat present low antigenicity and consequently lead to weak rejection; bone, muscles, nerves and vessels show a moderate rejection profile in spite of various degrees of immunogenicity; skin, a complex immunological structure, is the component which develops the most severe rejection because of the abundance of dentritic cells within epidermis and dermis. Finally, bone marrow, a source of immunocompetent cells, is a major target for rejection, but also a source of contaminating donor T cells that could induce a graft versus host disease in a strongly immunosuppressed recipient, and a source of stem cells that might contribute to the development of a microchimerism.

In humans few cases of isolated muscle [3], bone, joint [4, 5], nerve [6] or vascular allografts [7] have been reported. The first vascularized human hand was transplanted on September 23rd 1998 in Lyon [8], and it is summarized in the present report in which the immunosuppressive treatment used is discussed.

P. Cochat et al. (eds.), Immunosuppression under Trial, 145–151
©1999 Kluwer Academic Publishers.

Case report

A 48-year-old New Zealand man suffered a traumatic circular saw amputation of his right forearm in 1984. This was initially replanted but required reamputation in 1989 because of lack of function.

The patient refused anaesthetic or functional prosthesis, preferring to explore the literature and making himself available to units contemplating limb transplantation. He was informed of all the potential risks and his decision was taken in total autonomy after psychological evaluation. He underwent routine pretransplantation investigations and specific morphological and functional tests of his forearm stump.

The donor was a 41-year-old man who died from an intracerebral haematoma secondary to a skull fracture. He had the same blood group (0+) as the recipient, there were six HLA mismatches (A, B and DR), and the crossmatch was negative. The brachial artery was dissected free 3 cm above the elbow joint and cannulated, and the limb was irrigated with 500 ml UW solution at 4° C before being amputated a few centimeters above the elbow.

Under general anaesthesia coupled with the administration of a brachial block, the recipient's stump was prepared by dissecting and identifying all available muscles and neurovascular structures. At the same time, the graft anatomical structures were dissected and tagged. Replantation consisted of sequential bone fixation, arterial and venous anastomoses (ischemia time 750 min), nerve sutures, muscle and tendon connections and cutaneous sutures.

The patient (90 kg body weight) was given 500 units of heparin subcutaneously on the first day and low molecular heparin (Fraxiparine 300 units) for 10 days, then aspirin 150 mg/day. A wide spectrum antibiotic therapy was administered for 10 days. The immunosuppression induction protocol consisted of antithymocyte globulins (thymoglobuline® 75 mg/day for 10 days); tacrolimus (Prograf®) to maintain blood levels between 10 and 15 ng/ml during the first month, Mycophenolate Mofetil (Cellcept®) 2 g/day and steroids (prednisone), 250 mg on the first day and then rapidly tapered to 20 mg/day. Anti-CD25 monoclonal antibody was given on day 26 and day 100. Maintenance therapy included tacrolimus (serum levels between 5 and 10 ng/ml), Mycophenolate Mofetil (2 g/day), prednisone (20 mg at 3 months). Sulfadoxine pyrimethamine (Fansidar) was given to prevent *Pneumocystis carinii* pneumonia.

Physiotherapy was started 10 h postoperatively and performed twice a day for the entire follow-up period. Psychological support was offered once a day during the first three weeks, then twice weekly.

Skin biopsies were taken once a week from several areas and more frequently when rejection was suspected.

No surgical complications were encountered and wound healing was satisfactory, as was the take of skin autografts. The blood supply was excellent as demonstrated initially by the PO_2 saturation values in all fingers and later by scintigraphy. The patient's general condition always remained satisfactory.

Hyperglycaemia requiring insulin administration followed by oral hypo-glycaemia agents coincided with the initial high doses of steroids and tacrolimus. Serum creatinine increased in parallel with high tacrolimus levels and returned to normal values with drug dose reduction. A herpesvirus (HSV-1) infection occured 2 months post-transplantation and was successfully treated with acyclovir.

At 8 weeks post-transplantation, following a decrease in tacrolimus plasma levels, the skin demonstrated a mild disseminated erythema and histologically a major perivascular dermal infiltrate of mononuclear cells consistent with rejection. Tacrolimus as well as prednisone doses (20–40 mg/day) doses were increased; in addition topical immunosuppression was started using tacrolimus and clobetasol (Dermoval®) ointment twice a day. This regimen kept the rejection episode under control, and subsequent skin biopsies showed nearly normal dermis.

Although no microchimerism was demonstrated in the peripheral blood by DNA typing on day 85 and day 100, Cd1a-positive Langerhans cells of the recipient (expressing the recipient's own MHC class 1 HLA-A24 antigen) were demonstrated by double immunohistochemical labeling within the graft epidermis and hair follicles of the grafted forearm on day 85.

The rehabilitation program consisted of passive and active exercises as well as an early sensory re-education. At one day post-transplantation passive finger and wrist mobilization was started, with active mobility at 3 weeks postopera-tively. At 6 weeks, passive mobility of all joints below the elbow was achieved and active mobility was possible with and without visual control. At 100 days post-transplantation slight active flexion and extension of the wrist and long fingers occurred, indicating healing of the musculo-tendinous junctions.

Tinel's sign advanced 21 cm in the median nerve and 20 cm in the ulnar nerve, reaching the crease wrist. These surprising data have to be interpreted with caution in view of the subjective component of the test. The patient is currently trying to perform the thumb-index pinch despite the lack of sensation.

Discussion

The single most important obstacle currently preventing clinical application of limb transplantation is not the inability to restore function but rather the risks associated with the present lack of specific, safe and effective immunosup-pressive therapy [9]. Indeed it was assumed that the major risk was rejection for the composite structure of this graft. In addition, no permanent acceptance of fully mismatched skin allografts has been reported in the absence of tolerance. Therefore in this pioneer case we clearly made the choice of providing the patient with the most potent immunosuppressive regimen presently available, combining antibodies (anti-human thymocyte globulins, anti CD25 monoclonal antibodies), a calcineurin inhibitor (tacrolimus), a purine synthesis inhibitor (mycophenolate mofetil) and steroids. This drug combination proved to be efficient in the short term, as shown by the clinical outcome of the patient. One of the main difficulties with CTA is the lack of known criteria for acute rejection episodes. We relied on clinical symptoms, serum levels of C-reactive protein and skin biopsies. Only the latter proved to be a reliable indicator of dermal rejection and we cannot be sure that unnoticed low-grade or localized rejection episodes did not develop in other tissues. Foci of hyperfixation observed on bone scintigraphy at 3 months may represent minor focal rejection. The only episode of skin rejection was observed between 8 and 9 weeks post-transplantation when serum tacrolimus concentration dropped as a consequence of drug dose reduction because of renal toxicity. The rejection episode was reversed by an increase in steroid doses (from 20 to 40 mg/day) and topical application of immunosuppressive creams (tacrolimus, Clobetasol). The contribution of local versus systemic treatment is difficult to ascertain retrospectively.

The use of thymoglobulins as induction therapy was decided because we needed a potent lymphoablative agent with rapid action in view of the high risk of rejection [10]. Following a 10-day course at standard dosage, there was a complete disappearance of peripheral blood T cells for one month, with a progressive recovery during the second month, characterized by a predominance of NK cells (300/μl) and low CD4$^+$ (50/μl) and CD8+ (150–200/μl) cell counts. The patient did not produce antibodies against rabbit ATG, but free antilymphocyte antibodies in his plasma decreased rapidly within a week after treatment. For this reason we decided to use a CD25 antibody given at monthly intervals to ensure further protection.

The risks of lymphoablative therapies such as ATG, Cdw52 and total body irradiation include excessive destruction of peripheral T cell pools with defective reconstitution of naive T cells in adults and loss of heterogeneity in the T cell repertoire. The precise dose–effect relationship and optimal risk/benefit ratios according to ATG dosage remain to be determined. The risk of CD25 antibody is the transient expression of IL-2Rα chain by activated T cells, and the possible activation of CD25 cells, resulting in a lack of efficacy of the antibody.

The decision to use a potent immunosuppressive treatment was also based on data reported in the literature. In rodents, the first cases of long-term, rejection-free survival of rat limb allografts were reported when high dose CSA was administered [11, 12]. Other authors have noted early or delayed skin rejection in CSA-treated animals [13]. In addition, discontinuation of CSA administration resulted in rapid rejection of rat vascularized muscle allografts, peripheral nerves allografts and vascularized bone allografts [14, 15]. The use of more modern immunosuppressants has only modestly improved the results. High oral doses of tacrolimus allowed long-term allograft survival [16, 17] and Mycophenolate Mofetil was shown to both prevent and reverse acute rejection with concomitant drug-induced side effects [18, 19]. Long-term graft survival was also obtained by a combination of low dose CSA and low dose

Mycophenolate Mofetil with less toxicity [18]. In non-human primates, long-term partial or total hand allograft survival required high and toxic doses of Cyclosporine A, steroids and monoclonal antibodies [20–22].

In addition to efficacy, safety is the main goal of all immunosuppressive treatments in clinical transplantation. In this patient, drug toxic side effects were hyperglycemia and increased serum creatinine. Hyperglycemia required several days of insulin therapy and then it was well controlled by oral anti-diabetic drugs as well as by the concomitant reduction in tacrolimus and steroid doses. On two occasions, serum creatinine increased and returned to normal values when tacrolimus serum concentration decreased.

Infections and malignancy are the most severe complications of immunosuppression. In this case a herpesvirus infection occurred 2 months post-transplantation and it was easily reversed by acyclovir treatment.

The most common malignancies induced by immunosuppression are lymphoid tumors and skin cancers [23]. The risk of EBV-associated B cell lymphoid tumor development is difficult to predict when a combination of new immunosuppressive drugs are combined with polyclonal or monoclonal antibodies. In the CTR Opelz reported a 0.28% incidence of lymphomas in patients treated with cyclosporin A and azathioprine. The risk of skin cancer is dramatically higher in Australia where it reaches up to 40 % of patients after 10 years of immunosuppressive treatment [24]. Reduction in sun exposure and ultraviolet filter creams as well as early detection and treatment of the lesions are adequate for prevention and therapy of this severe complication.

In the present case topical application of FK506 and Clobetasol creams were used in the prevention and/or the treatment of the rejection episode. The main advantage of the local drug administration is to deliver locally a sufficient amount of immunosuppressive drugs without increasing their serum levels and consequent toxicity [25]. Other investigators developed several CTA models of immunosuppression, such as intra-arterial infusion and liposomes [26]. Preliminary results are controversial and further studies are needed to determine the efficacy of a local immunosuppressive therapy [9]. Although chronic administration of immunosuppressive agents is accepted in visceral organ transplantation, the risks associated with such treatment in patients requiring a functional non-vital part of the body should be discussed. In our opinion, the recipient is the only person able to make an appropriate decision after a complete information on the graft and the immunosuppressive treatment.

In conclusion, in absence of further rejection this CTA case opens one of the last frontiers in clinical transplantation.

Acknowledgments

We thank J.J. Colpart Regional Coordinator of the Etablissement Français des Greffes and his team, G. Burloux (psychology), C. Frances (dermatology), G. Herzberg, M. Lanzetta, H. Kapila, V. Guigal, G. Pasticier, L. Pibiri, N. Courtois (surgery), D. Mongin-Long, C. Kopp, A. Ostapetz (Anesthesiology), D. Lyonnet, M. Bochu (radiology), J. M. Ramackers (scintigraphy), M.P. Auboyer, procedure coordinator and finally Charles Merieux and the Merieux Foundation for their generous support.

References

1. Llull R. An open proposal for clinical composite tissue allotransplantation. Transplant. Proc. 1998, 30: 2692–2696.
2. Graham B, Adkins P, Tsai TM, Firell J, Breidenbach WC. Major replantation versus revision amputation and prosthetic fitting in the upper extremity: a late functional outcomes study. J. Hand Surg. 1998; 23A: 783–791.
3. Jones TR, Humphrey PA, Brennan DC. Transplantation of vascularized allogeneic skeletal muscle for scalp reconstruction in a renal transplant patient. Transplant. Proc. 1998; 30: 2746–2753.
4. Hofmann GO, Kirschner MH, Wagner FD, Brauns L, Gonschorek O, Buhren V. Allogeneic vascularized transplantation of human femoral diaphyses and total knee joint – first clinical experiences. Transplant. Proc. 1998; 30: 2754–2761.
5. Guimberteau JC, Baudet J, Panconi B, Boileau R, Potaux I. Human allotransplant of a digital flexion system vascularized on the ulnar pedicle: a preliminary report and 1-year follow-up of two cases. Plast. Reconstr. Surg. 1992; 89: 1137–1147.
6. Mackinnon SE, Hudson AL. Clinical application of peripheral nerve transplantation. Plast. Reconstr. Surg. 1992; 90: 695–699.
7. Carpenter JP, Tomaszewski JP. Immunosuppression for human saphenous vein allografts by pass surgery a prospective randomized trial. J. Vasc. Surg. 1997; 26: 32–42.
8. Dubernard JM, Owen ER, Herzberg G et al. Human hand allograft: report on the first six months. Lancet. 1999; April 17: 1315–1320.
9. Shirbachech MV, Jones JW, Breidenbach WC, McCabes, Barker JH and Gruber SA. The case for local immunosuppression in composite tissue allotransplantation. Transplant. Proc. 1998; 30: 2739–2742.
10. Revillard JP, Bonnefoy-Berard N, Preville X et al. Immunopharmacology of thymoglobulin (ATG). GRAFT, 1999; 2: 177–180.
11. Black KS, Hewitt CV, Fraser LA, Howard EB, Martin DC, Achauer BM, Furnas DW. Composite tissue (limb) allografts in rats. II. Indefinite survival using low-dose cyclosporine. Transplantation. 1985; 39: 365–368.
12. Black KS, Hewitt CV, Hwang JS. Transdermal application of Cyclosporine prolongs skin allograft survival. Transplant. Proc. 1988; 20: 660–662.
13. Benhaim P, Anthony JP, Lin LY, McCalmont TH, Mathes SJ. A long term study of allogeneic rat hindlimb transplants immunosuppressed with RS-61443. Transplantation. 1993; 56: 911–917.
14. Yeh LS, Gregory CR, Griffey SM, Lecouteur RA, Morris RE. Results of Leflunomide and Cyclosporine on myocutaneous allograft survival in the rat. Transplantation. 1996; 62: 861–863.
15. Yeh LS, Gregory CR, Griffey SM, Lecouteur RA, Hou SM, Morris RE. Combination leflunomide and Cyclosporine prevents rejection of functional whole limb allografts in the rat. Transplantation. 1997; 64: 919–922.
16. Fealy MJ, Umansky WS, Bicjel KD, Nino JJ, Morris RE, Press BH. Efficacy of rapamycin and FK 506 in prolonging rat hind limb allograft survival. Ann. Surg. 1994; 219: 88–93.
17. Fealy MJ, Most D, Huie P, Wolf M, Sibley RK, Morris RE, Press BH. Association of down-regulation of cytokine activity with rat hind limb allograft survival. Transplantation. 1995; 59: 1475–1480.
18. Benhaim P, Antony JP, Ferreira L, Borsanyi JP, Mathes SJ. Use of combination of low dose cyclosporine and RS61443 in a rat hindlimb model of composite tissue allotransplantation.

Transplantation. 1996; 61: 527–532.

19. Van Den Helder TB, Benhaim P, Anthony JP, McCalmont TH, Mathes SJ. Efficacy of RS - 61443 in reversing acute rejection in a rat model of hindlimb allotransplantation. Transplantation. 1994; 57: 427–433.
20. Skanes SE, Samulak DD, Daniel RK. Tissue transplantation for reconstructive surgery. Transplant. Proc. 1986; 18: 898–900.
21. Stark GB, Swartz WM, Narayanan K, Moller AR. Hand transplantation in baboons. Transplant. Proc. 1987; 19: 3968–3971.
22. Stevens HP, Hovius SE, Heney HT. Immunologic aspects and complications of composite tissue allografting for upper extremity reconstruction: a study in the rhesus monkey. Transplant. Proc. 1991; 23: 623–625.
23. First MR, Peddi VR. Malignancies complicating organ transplantation. Transplant. Proc. 1998; 30: 2768–2770.
24. Digiovanna JJ. Postransplantation skin cancer: scope of the problem, management and role for systemic retenoid dermoprevention. Transplant. Proc. 1998, 30: 2771–2775.
25. Yuzawa K, Taniguchi H, Seino K, Otsuka, Fukao K. Topical immunosuppression in skin grafting with FK506 ointment. Transplant. Proc. 1996; 28: 1387–1389.
26. Ko S, Nakajima Y, Kanerhiro. The enhanced immunosuppressive efficacy of newly developed liposomal FK 506 in canine liver transplantation. Transplantation. 1995; 59: 1384–1388.

18. The search for immunosuppressive synergy

C. VAN BUREN

The dramatic growth in the armamentarium of immunosuppressive agents available to the practicing transplant surgeon or physician has created a new set of challenges. How does one determine the optimum regimen? What is the *sine qua non* of new breakthrough agent? How can one rationally establish a protocol that will balance efficacy of therapy with cost-effectiveness? The answers to these questions can determine the success in attracting new patients as well as the financial well-being of a transplant center.

The traditional approach has been to adopt each new agent that is developed and to add it to the therapeutic protocol. The first example of such an approach was the use of cyclosporine. Most transplant programs added this agent to the immunosuppressive agents azathioprine and corticosteroids to maintain transplant patients. Cyclosporine was the most costly part of the regimen, but clearly resulted in significantly improved one year graft survival, a 50% reduction in treated rejection rates, and a reduction in opportunistic infections. One could quibble that controlled studies failed to document that azathioprine in combination with prednisone and cyclosporine improved graft survival compared to cyclosporine-steroid regimens alone, but the cost of azathioprine was relatively low.

The 'onion approach', the therapeutic strategy which added another layer of immunosuppression on to the underlying layers in the therapeutic protocol when a new agent was developed, began to demonstrate the limitation of the approach when examining the role of T-lymphocyte xenoantibody preparations. These regimens may improve graft survival by 2–5%, although no controlled studies document this efficacy. Rejection rates are moderately lower. However, complication rates including cytomegalovirus (CMV) infections and lympho-proliferative disorders are dramatically higher. To decrease the risk of CMV infections, gangcyclovir is added to the regimen. In addition, monitoring both of lymphocyte subsets to document efficacy and for anti-mouse or anti-horse antibodies, depending on the xenoantibodies used, also add to the cost. One is confronted by an increase of $6,000 to $8,000 in pharmacy and monitoring costs to realize little improvement in graft survival. To avoid this dilemma drug synergy is sought if one is to maximize the benefit derived and to minimize the cost expended, both financially and in incidence of complications.

P. Cochat et al. (eds.), Immunosuppression under Trial,, 153–155
©1999 Kluwer Academic Publishers.

Another reason to explore for synergistic interactions between immuno-suppressive agents is to minimize drug induced side effects. Cyclosporine or FK506 nephrotoxicity is a complication that leads to a reduction in the dose of calcineurin inhibitors as a part of many therapeutic protocols. However, both of these agents have poor bioavailability. Moreover, intra-individual variability in drug absorption has been documented to be associated with increased rejection and poorer allograft survival. Thus, a synergistic interaction between cyclosporine and newer immunosuppressants will in a dependable fashion both decrease complications of nephrotoxicity and potentially avoid the problem of dropping the drug dose below the therapeutic window in order to minimize side effects.

With the rapidly expanding choices of new agents in study or recently released for clinical use, one needs a rational means of choosing which agent will be most cost effective. The mathematical model for such a reason-based definition of a therapeutic protocol was derived from the field of clinical oncology, where a wide array of chemotherapeutic agents are available for the practicing oncologist. In this formula, the combination index or C.I. is calculated based on dose response curves of drugs used individually or in combination using the following formula:

$$\text{C.I.} = \frac{D_1 \text{ combined}}{D_1 \text{ alone}} + \frac{D_2 \text{ combined}}{D_2 \text{ alone}}$$

where D represents dosed of drugs which result in 50% of maximal putative response.

Once these determinations have been made in the animal laboratory, appropriate doses of immunosuppressives can be calculated for initial trials to test toxicity and later efficacy.

An example of an additive agent is mycophenolate mofetil (MMF), an S-phase agent that additively improves experimental allograft survival when combined with cyclosporine. Clinical studies document that MMF reduced treated rejection episodes by 50%, but does not improve allograft survival. If the underlying incidence of treated rejection episodes is 40% at a given clinical transplant center, the cost of treating 100% of patients with MMF will have to be less than the cost savings in the 20% of patients that will not suffer rejection. The problems with justifying the use of such an agent on the basis of cost savings becomes apparent.

Furthermore, elimination of agents such as corticosteroids, which are synergistic when combined with cyclosporine, becomes less likely, based on using an agent such as MMF whose effect is only additive. Thus, based on this reasoning, the failure of the multicenter steroid withdrawal study in MMF-cyclosporine treated patients, could perhaps have been anticipated.

In contrast, the macrolide rapamycin, is genuinely synergistic with cyclosporine in experimental studies. Clinical trials document both a 75% reduction in rejection episodes as well as an improved survival of primary cadaveric allografts. The use of a synergistic agent such as rapamycin offers the opportunity to save cost by reducing the use of cyclosporine, to reduce drug induced nephrotoxicity, and to avoid the morbid side effects of the cortico- steroids which are also synergistic with cyclosporine.

These considerations are examples of how documented synergy between drugs can lead to rational programs that implement new immunosuppressive technologies that emerge based upon cost-benefit analysis or predictable decrease in complications.

19. Economic analysis of immunosuppression in transplantation: a review of recent studies in liver and kidney transplantation

J. HUTTON

Introduction

Organ transplantation has been widely recognized as the preferred approach, both clinically and economically, to the management of severe disease in several organs of the human body. In spite of the high initial cost of the surgical procedures the extensive patient benefits make such interventions a cost-effective use of health care resources. In many situations, such as chronic heart disease or liver failure, there is no other treatment which can ensure patient survival, so the benefit of transplantation comes in the form of years of life gained. In other organs, such as the kidney, alternative approaches exist which can prolong life. However, the quality of life of patients on dialysis can be much worse than for those with a successful transplant, so significant patient benefits come in the form of quality-adjusted life years which combine the gain in length and quality of life.

Renal transplantation has received more attention from economists than other types of transplantation. One of the earliest examples of economic evaluation in health care was of renal transplantation [1]. Several subsequent studies have confirmed its cost effectiveness [2–4]. In spite of this strong economic and clinical support, renal transplantation cannot be made available to all end-stage renal disease (ESRD) patients who might benefit from the procedure because of a shortage of donor organs. Consequently, it is necessary to ensure efficient use of those donor organs which are available, by minimizing chronic rejection and the need for retransplantation. The key element in this is the immunosuppressive treatment given to the patient. Considerable investment in research and development has led to a significant number of new products reaching or about to reach the market. Clinicians are now faced with a range of options and combinations from which to choose. As the price of the individual products varies considerably, it is essential to have a full picture of the total impact on heath care resource use as well as the clinical impact of the drugs.

P. Cochat et al. (eds.), Immunosuppression under Trial, 157–166
©1999 Kluwer Academic Publishers.

Main economic factors

The clinical and economic issues surrounding immunosuppression are common to most organ transplant procedures. This review will concentrate on renal and liver transplantation as there is a more extensive literature on the economics of immunosuppression in these areas. The cost effectiveness of the main transplantation procedure in liver and kidney compares favourably with that of many other health care interventions [5]. Successful transplantation involves a high initial cost of obtaining the donor organ, carrying out the grafting operation and managing complications and acute rejection episodes (which are concentrated in the first year post-transplant). Subsequent graft failure raises the possibility of the need for retransplantation or reversion to dialysis in the case of ESRD. The more successful the immunosuppression treatment in extending patient and graft survival the more cost effective it is likely to be. Economic comparisons of different approaches to managing ESRD and liver failure should ideally cover the full expected lifetime of the patients. This ensures that the full survival and quality of life benefit is captured as well as the changing cost profile over time.

Improving the transplantation process

While the general case for use of transplantation, where possible, has been well established in economic terms, the selection of variants in the immunosuppression regime used in conjunction with transplantation is less clear cut. There are three main stages to the immunosuppression treatment: induction therapy prior to transplantation; the immediate post-transplantation phase in which a combination of therapies is usually used; and the maintenance phase in which the patient is stabilized on lower doses of the main immunosuppressive drug. When acute rejection episodes occur they are managed by increased doses of some therapeutic agents (e.g. steroids) or by rescue therapy with another immunosuppressive drug. This may lead to a permanent switch of the main immunosuppressive agent. Drugs may also be changed as a result of adverse events or lack of patient tolerance.

The short-term success of the immunosuppressive therapy is assessed in terms of the avoidance of acute rejection episodes and adverse events. The management of these may require rehospitalization as well as the use of more expensive rescue therapies. There is also some evidence of lower perceived quality of life in patients suffering acute rejection episodes in the first year after transplantation, in comparison with those with no rejection [6]. The long-term success of immunosuppression is indicated by the avoidance of chronic rejection, graft failure and the need for a possible retransplantation. In the worst cases of chronic rejection patient survival will be affected if no organ is available for retransplantation. For ESRD patients successful immunosuppression avoids the long-term costs and loss of quality of life associated with dialysis.

Economic comparisons

In comparing immunosuppressive treatments it is necessary to consider the long-term benefits in terms of extended patient survival and improved quality of life, as well as the short-term resource savings which may result from avoidance of acute rejection episodes and adverse events. More expensive immunosuppressive agents, for example induction therapy with antibodies, may offset much of their extra cost through avoidance of the costs of managing acute rejections, such as rehospitalization, short-term dialysis, and rescue therapy. After stabilization of patients in the first year acute phase, the overall cost of medications, including maintenance immunosuppressive agents, should be evaluated against the cost of long-term complications. These can include graft failure which requires a retransplantation or a return to dialysis in the case of ESRD patients.

The cost framework alone is insufficient to cover all the relevant economic variables so analysis is best conducted in terms of cost effectiveness or cost–utility analysis [7]. This allows the gain in patient survival and improvements in quality of life to be assessed against the costs of achieving them. Therapies which add to the direct drug cost can be preferred if they produce additional social benefits in sufficient quantities.

The most powerful economic case can be made if a link can be established between better short-term outcomes, such as reduction of acute rejection episodes, and better long-term outcomes, such as improved graft survival.

Data for economic analysis

There are two main approaches to the collection of data for economic evaluations of drugs. One method is to collect data on health care resource use, and relevant economic outcomes such as quality of life and utility, in the course of a clinical trial. This gives a measure of the resources used to achieve any differences in outcomes observed in the trial. The alternative approach is to use a decision modeling framework and bring together data from a variety of sources. In practice a combination of both approaches is necessary. The main advantage of the trial-based approach is that the data are collected prospectively and patients have been randomized to treatments. However, the duration of trials is rarely long enough to observe the long-term differences in outcomes. This is true in the immunosuppression field where trials rarely last more than 2 years but long-term outcome differences may take up to 10 years to emerge. If there are known clinical indicators which are predictive of long-term outcomes, than these can be modeled using the trial data as a base.

Trials can be used to collect major items of resource use such as hospitalizations and use of drugs in a reliable way. The more detailed recording of resource use in the management of rejection episodes and adverse events may be more difficult. It is often easier to observe the frequency of these clinical events in a trial and to carry out a separate exercise in parallel to estimate the cost of managing each type of rejection episode and adverse event [8].

Studies in liver and renal transplantation have used each of these approaches, although most have concentrated on the short-term impact of immunosuppressive therapies.

Comparative economic evaluations: renal transplantation

Cyclosporin versus tacrolimus

Until recently the main immunosuppressive agent used in renal transplantation was cyclosporin A. This is usually combined with azathioprine and corticosteroids in the immediate post-transplantation period. A newer immunosuppressive agent, tacrolimus (FK506), has been introduced which has been shown to reduce the frequency of acute rejection in renal transplantation when compared with cyclosporin [9].

Several economic evaluations have been carried out based on short-term data from trials comparing tacrolimus and cyclosporin in Europe and the US. Olivera reported a study of the cost savings from the prevention of acute rejections in the UK, based on 1 year data from the European Multicentre Study [10]. Frequency of acute rejections was taken from the trial data and resource use and costs were estimated separately for each type of rejection. Although there was no significant difference in the overall healthcare costs for the tacrolimus and cyclosporin arms of the trial, the acute rejection costs per patient in the tacrolimus arm were one-third of those in the cyclosporin arm. The study did not assess any gain in quality of life from avoidance of rejection episodes which would accrue to patients on tacrolimus.

An economic assessment based on the US multicenter randomized trial of tacrolimus and cyclosporin [11] compared hospitalization costs for the two arms of the study [12]. The mean costs of the initial hospitalization were similar for the two groups, but rehospitalized patients had a longer average length of stay in the cyclosporin group and their total rehospitalization costs were higher.

Once the patient is stabilized on maintenance immunosuppression, which is usually the case after the first year post-transplantation, there are no longer any savings from the avoidance of acute rejections and adverse events. Net savings would occur only if there was a sufficiently large difference in the early graft failure rate for the consequent costs of retransplantation and reversion to dialysis, which would be avoided by the more successful drug.

In the case of tacrolimus and cyclosporin such differences in early graft failure were not observed but evidence emerging from 3 year follow-up in the US study indicates that the long-term effectiveness of tacrolimus is maintained [13]. Graft survival at 3 years was 82.4% for tacrolimus and 79.2% for cyclosporin. When cross-overs for rejection in the trial were counted as graft failures the figures were 81.5% and 70% respectively. Evidence from cohort studies also indicates that the longer term differences may increase. Gjertson and colleagues [14] followed-up first cadaveric renal transplants in 38057 patients for 3 years. The respective graft survival rates for tacrolimus and cyclosporin patients were 92% and 86%. Extrapolation of first year survival data (i.e. patients with a surviving graft at 1 year) estimated a graft half-life of 14.1 years for tacrolimus patients and 9.1 years for the cyclosporin group [15]. If these figures are confirmed then the implication is that the cyclosporin group will incur the extra cost of return to dialysis or retransplantation 5 years sooner. Using these projections an economic evaluation was carried out by Booth-Clibborn and colleagues relating to the UK [16]. The cost of maintenance immunosuppression with tacrolimus was more than offset by the cost of returning to haemodialysis 5 years earlier. The long term savings for tacrolimus were estimated to be £89000 per patient.

Cyclosporin microemulsion

To overcome problems associated with inconsistent absorption of cyclosporin, a new formulation, has been developed which forms a microsuspension on contact with gastrointestinal fluids. This reduces the variability of blood cyclosporin levels and may reduce the incidence of acute rejection. Two preliminary economic studies have been published comparing the microemulsion with the older cyclosporin formulation in Canada [17, 18]. These studies did not produce any statistically significant cost differences, although there were some trends in favour of the new formulation. The lack of significant differences was not surprising since the studies lasted only 12 weeks and enrolled 30 and 41 patients respectively. A further study in Europe which followed 68 patients in three countries for 12 months has been partially reported. From both the health insurance and the societal perspectives, potential savings from the use of the new formulation were identified when compared with Sandimmun [19].

The above studies were adjuncts to clinical trials and although the data were collected prospectively the studies were not primarily designed to test economic hypotheses. They are of limited use as they do not compare the cyclosporin microemulsion with any of the newer immunosuppressants. A recent UK study, using a retrospective design, analyzed resources used in the management of adult cadaveric renal transplant patients with either Neoral or tacrolimus as primary immunosuppression [20]. Eighty-nine patients with at least 6 months of follow-up were included. Mean costs per patient were similar at £13200 for Neoral and £12982 for tacrolimus patients. These results are similar to the one year studies comparing cyclosporin and tacrolimus referred to above.

Antibodies

Antilymphocyte products are used for induction therapy in some transplant centres, mainly antithymocyte globulin (ATG) and muromonab CD3 (OKT3).

ATG costs more than OKT3 but the latter may have more severe side-effects. Shield et al. [21] compared the costs of induction therapy with OKT3 with no induction therapy, by modeling clinical trial results and financial data from separate sources. They concluded that the extra costs of the OKT3 would be offset by savings in other costs resulting from the lower acute rejection rate. Schommer et al. [22] compared the costs of ATG and OKT3 in a retrospective, multicentre study using charge data. The increased pharmacy charges for ATG were partially offset by reductions in ancillary charges. However, the variations in clinical practice and charging policies at different centres made interpretation of the results difficult.

Brennan et al. [23] carried out a retrospective study in a single centre, of 183 patients receiving induction therapy with either ATG or OKT3 between 1991 and 1994. The one year post-transplant rejection rate was lower for ATG , 13% versus 34% for OKT3 and graft survival was better in the ATG group. These clinical advantages translated into a trend towards lower overall hospital-related costs for ATG, $39,937 ± 17,014 as against $42,850 ± 20,923. Although not statistically significant, the economic results of this study can be related to the clinical differences, and the outcome and economic data come from the same patient group.

New products

Economic evidence has recently become available about another new immuno-suppressive agent mycophenolate mofetil (MMF). In an evaluation based on clinical trial data Sullivan et al. compared the costs of quadruple therapies involving induction, cyclosporine, corticosteroids and MMF or azathioprine in the first year after transplant [24]. The results show that on average the patients treated with MMF will have a lower incidence of rejection, better graft survival and no difference in opportunistic infections. This leads to slightly lower first year treatment costs with MMF because the higher immunosuppression cost is more than offset by the lower rejection-related treatment costs and the lower dialysis and graft failure costs. In a similar study from the Canadian perspective the result was reversed with the MMF treatment group having slightly higher costs [25], indicating the sensitivity of the comparison to differences in practice patterns and relative costs of health care resources.

Comparative evaluations: liver transplantation

The literature on the cost effectiveness of immunosuppression in liver transplantation is not as extensive as that for kidney. Several studies of the comparative costs of the older and newer formulations of cyclosporin and reviewed by Coukell and Plasker [26]. Many of these studies have been published only as abstracts, and although many show trends towards cost savings from the use of the microemulsion formulation, none reach statistical significance. For example, a prospective resource utilisation study based on the MILTON trial indicated a trend towards 8–10% cost savings in the 4 month post-transplant period [27].

Cost comparison of tacrolimus and cyclosporin in the US have shown cost savings from the reduced rate of acute rejections with tacrolimus [28]. The European multicentre clinical trial showed that in liver transplantation tacrolimus is associated with a significant reduction in acute, refractory acute and chronic rejection episodes compared with cyclosporin [29]. An economic analysis based on 2 year post-transplant data from the trial showed 15% higher costs for the cyclosporin patients, a result that proved robust in extensive sensitivity analysis [30].

Quality of life and utility

Formal assessment of quality of life and utility has not formed a major part of outcomes assessment in economic evaluations of immunosuppression regimes in transplantation. Several earlier studies addressed the quality of life of renal transplant patients per se [31] and the recent study by Shield et al. [6] has confirmed the difference in quality of life between transplanted patients and those on dialysis. This study also showed a negative impact on quality of life from the incidence of acute rejections. Keown et al. [25] calculate costs per quality-adjusted life year gained in the first year post-transplant from the use of MMF at CD$50717. The methodology is not explained in the abstract.

Booth-Clibborn et al. [16] estimated utilities for the health states associated with rejection episodes using the Index of Health-related Quality of Life (IHQL). Using these values they estimate the short-term (first year) utility gains from using tacrolimus instead of cyclosporin to accrue at a rate in excess of £120000 per QALY. This assumes no benefit other than reduced incidence of rejection episodes and that benefits do not last beyond the first year. However, using the data on projected graft survival differences, and the utilities for having a successful graft as opposed to being on dialysis, their analysis over the longer term shows a significant gain in QALYs and a cost saving of £75000 per QALY gained.

The above studies differentiate between treatments on the basis of differences in clinical outcomes such as rejection rates and graft survival which have been shown to have an impact on quality of life regardless of the treatment being given. The only quality of life study which differentiates between immunosuppressive regimes on the basis of product-specific side effects is that by Shield et al. [6]. In this study a statistically significant difference between patients on tacrolimus and those on cyclosporin was found in the Bergner Physical Appearance scale. This was a separate scale specifically designed to measure the quality of life impact of side effects such as gingival hyperplasia and facial hirsutism. An isolated result of this kind is difficult to interpret without knowledge of the importance of these factors in overall quality of life.

Discussion

The literature on economic outcomes of different immunosuppression regimes in transplantation is small but growing. As new and more expensive treatments are added to the available products the need to demonstrate consequent resource savings as well as clinical benefits is being increasingly recognized. Most of the analyses so far published have concentrated on the first year post-transplant in which the impact of variable acute rejection rates and side-effect profiles is felt. Statistically significant differences in graft survival are not seen at this stage in clinical trials, so it is not surprising that significant economic differences have not been observed. Most studies of this type show that the costs of many immunosuppression regimes are similar, with the higher costs of newer therapies being offset by treatment cost savings resulting from their short-term efficacy.

The value of some of these studies is limited by small sample sizes in trial-based studies, and retrospective data collection methodologies. Use of clinical records from case series can provide a good representation of resource use in routine practice but does not provide the most reliable evidence of comparative clinical effects of drugs. The best economic analyses have used larger clinical trials for the efficacy and resource use data, and supplemented these from other sources to complete the cost analysis.

Comparison of results is difficult because of the differences in the way costs have been calculated. Brennan et al. [23] and Morris-Stiff et al. [20] included the costs of the transplant procedure in the first year costs while Olivera [10] included the initial hospitalization but not the transplant procedure. Keown et al. [17] and Sullivan et al. [24] excluded both, while Kingma et al. [18] excluded the transplant procedure and are unclear on the treatment of the initial hospitalization.

Economic analyses restricted to one year post-transplant are of limited value in determining the ultimate impact of improved immunosuppression therapy. Comparative observational data is not available in the long-term to facilitate lifetime economic analysis for renal or liver transplant patients. There is always least information on the most recent drug, making projection and modelling of outcomes essential. Exploratory analyses such as that of Booth-Clibborn and colleagues [16] indicate the extreme importance of taking the long-term view and having accurate empirical measures of utilities. If the results of that study are confirmed by subsequent work, the potential economic benefits of new immunosuppressants with superior performance to cyclosporin could be very great.

The current literature does not give a clear picture of the relative cost effectiveness of the different immunosuppressants since the full range of comparisons has not been included in clinical trials. Many new agents have been compared with regimes containing the older formulation of cyclosporin rather than the new microemulsion formulation. Economic studies of the new formulation have only compared it with the older formulation of cyclosporin. A recent comprehensive review of the economic literature on the use of the new microemulsion formulation of cyclosporin concluded that published studies 'showed a consistent, although small and not statistically significant, reduction in cost associated with (its) use' in comparison with the older formulation. Studies have also shown cost reductions from the use of tacrolimus in comparison with the older cyclosporin, but no studies have compared it directly with the new formulation as yet. The economic benefit of different antibody induction regimens and other combinations of immunosuppressents, in comparison with more standard approaches, cannot be judged from the limited number of restricted evaluation studies currently published. With the variations of induction therapy, and alternatives to azathioprine now available to combine with cyclosporin or tacrolimus, the immediate need for economic data can only be met by modeling studies. By using the best information currently available on rejection rates, graft survival, immunosuppression costs and utilities, such studies could help to clarify the current state of knowledge and identify the important empirical questions to be answered in future cost–effectiveness trials.

Acknowledgements

The research on which this paper is based was partly funded by a grant from Fujisawa SA to MEDTAP International. The sections on renal transplantation are based on a paper previously published in *Transplantation Proceedings* [32]. The author would like to thank his colleagues Florian Hollenbach and Michael McKenna for research assistance and Annette Brady for assistance in manuscript preparation.

References

1. Klarman HF, Francis JO, Rosenthal CD. Cost-effectiveness analysis applied to the treatment of chronic renal diseases. Med. Care. 1968; 6: 48–54.
2. Ludbrook A. A cost-effectiveness analysis of the treatment of chronic renal failure. App. Econ. 1981; 13: 340–350.
3. Evans RW. The socioeconomics of organ transplantation. Transplant. Proc. 1985; 17 (Suppl 4): 129–136.
4. Karlberg I, Nyberg G. Cost-effectiveness studies of renal transplantation. Int. J. Tech. Ass. Health Care. 1995; 11: 611–622.
5. Maynard AK. Developing the health care market. Econ. J. 1991; 101: 1277.
6. Shield CF, McGrath MM, Gross TF. Assessment of health-related quality of life in kidney transplant receiving tacrolimus (FK507) based versus cyclosporine-based immunosuppression. Transplantation. 1997; 64: 1738–1743.
7. Drummond MF, Jefferson TO. Guidelines for peer reviewers and authors of economic submissions to the BMJ. BMJ. 1996; 313: 275–283.
8. Buxton MJ, Drummond MF, van Hout BA et al. Modelling in economic evaluation: an unavoidable fact of life. Health Econ. 1997; 6: 217–227.
9. European Tacrolimus Multi Centre Renal Study Group. Multicentre trial comparing tacrolimus (FK507) and cyclosporin in the prevention of renal allograft rejection: a report of the European Tacrolimus Multicentre Renal Study Group. Transplantation. 1997; 64: 436–443.

10. Olivera D. Economic analysis of Prograf® (tacrolimus) and cyclosporin in the prevention of kidney allograft rejection. New Horizons Kidney Transplant. 1997; 1: 12–15.
11. Pirsch JD, Miller J, Deierhoi MH et al. A comparison of tacrolimus (FK506) and cyclosporin for immunosuppression after cadaveric renal transplantation. Transplantation. 1997; 63: 977–983.
12. Neylan JF, FK506 Kidney Transplant Study Group, Sullivan EM et al. An economic assessment of post-transplant hospitalisations among kidney transplant patients receiving tacrolimus versus cyclosporine immunosuppressive therapy. ASTP Meeting Orlando, Florida 11013 Dec, 1997. Abstracts No. 100.
13. Jensik SC. Tacrolimus in Kidney transplantation: 3 year survival results of the US multicentre randomised comparative study. ASTP Meeting, Orlando, Florida 11–13 Dec 1997; Abstract No. 156.
14. Gjertson DW, Cecka JM, Terasaki PI. The relative effects of FK506 and cyclosporine on short- and long-term kidney graft survival. Transplantation. 1995; 60: 1384–1388.
15. Gjertson DW, Cecka JM, Terasaki PI. Long-term effect of Prograf on kidney graft survival. United Network for Organ Sharing, 1996.
16. Booth-Clibborn N, Best L, Stein K. Tacrolimus after kidney transplantation. DEC Report No 74, NHS Executive South and West. R&D Directorate, 1997.
17. Keown P, Lawen JG, Landsberg D et al. Economic analysis of Sandimmune Neoral in Canada in stable renal transplant patients. Transplant. Proc. 1995; 27: 1845–1848.
18. Kingma I, Ludwin D, Dandavion R et al. Economic analysis of Neoral in de novo renal transplantation. Clin. Transplant. 1997; 11; 42–48.
19. Abella I. Pharmacoeconomics of Neoral, a new formulation of cyclosporine, in renal transplantation. Transplant. Proc. 1996; 28: 3131–3134.
20. Morris-Stiff G, Richards T, Singh J et al. Pharmacoeconomic study of FK506 (Prograf) and cyclosporine A (Neoral) in cadaveric renal transplantation. Transplant. Proc. 1998; 30: 1285–1286.
21. Shield CF, Jacobs JR, Wyant S et al. A cost effectiveness analysis of OKT3 induction therapy in cadaveric kidney transplantation. Am. J. Kidney Dis. 1996; 27: 855–864.
22. Schommer JC, Pleil AM, Pathak DS. Two approaches to comparing hospital charges between cadaveric renal transplant patients who received OKT3 sterile solution or ATGAM sterile solution for induction therapy. Clin. Ther. 1995; 17: 749–769.
23. Brennan DC, Schnitzler MA, Baty JD et al. A pharmacoeconomic comparison of anti-thymocyte globulin and muromonab CD3 induction therapy in renal transplant recipients. Pharmacoeconomics. 1997; 11: 237–245.
24. Sullivan SD, Garrison LP, Best JH et al. The cost-effectiveness of mycophenolate mofetil in the first year after primary cadaveric transplant. J. Am. Soc. Nephrol. 1997; 8: 1592–1598.
25. Keown P, Sullivan SD, Best JH et al. Economic evaluation of mycophenolate mofetil (MMF) for prevention of acute graft rejection after cadaveric renal transplantation in Canada. ASTP Meeting Orlando, Florida 11–13 Dec 199. Abstract.
26. Coukell AJ, Plasker GL. Cyclosporin microemulsion (Neoral): a pharmacoeconomic review of its use compared with standard cyclosporin in renal and hepatic transplantation. Pharmacoeconomics. 1998; 14: 691–708.
27. Peeters P, Kazek M, Abella I et al. Economic evaluation of Neoral versus sandimmune main-tenance therapy for de novo liver transplant patients: results from an international randomized controlled trial. Transplant. Proc. 1998; 30: 1838–1842.
28. Lake JR, Gorman KJ, Esquirel CO et al. A cost comparison of liver transplantation with FK506 and CyA as the primary immunosuppression agent. Transplantation. 1995; 60: 1089–1095.
29. European FK506 Multicentre Liver Study Group. Randomized trial comparing tacrolimus (FK506) and cyclosporine in prevention of liver allograft rejection. Lancet. 1994; 344: 423–428.
30. McKenna M, Alexander G, Jones M, Hutton J. Economic analysis of tacrolimus (FK506) and cyclosporine in prevention of liver allograft rejection. Eur. Hosp. Pharm. 1996; 2: 181–188.
31. Evans RG, Hart G, Manninen DL. A comparative assessment of the quality of life of successful kidney transplant patients according to source of graft. Transplant. Proc. 1994; 16: 1353.
32. Hutton J. The economics of immunosuppression in renal transplantation: a review of recent literature. Transplant. Proc. 1999; 31: 1328–1332.

PART SIX

Clinical trials for at-risk situations

20. Questions raised by the exclusion of 'at risk' conditions from current trials in organ transplantation

J. P. REVILLARD, C. POUTEIL-NOBLE and P. COCHAT

Introduction

The recent development of new immunosuppressive agents may improve the overall results of organ transplantation and open new areas for clinical applications of allografts. The introduction of cyclosporin A 20 years ago brought drastic improvements in liver and heart transplantation, and these became routine treatment for irreversible hepatic or cardiac failure. New immunosuppressors may have a comparable effect on lung, heart–lung and intestinal transplantation. However the whole clinical field of organ transplantation is moving: improvement in short-term results has led to such treatments being offered to 'high-risk' patients who were formerly excluded from transplantation: carefully designed clinical studies demonstrated that very young or elderly recipients, as well as diabetics or hyperimmunized patients could benefit from such treatments. Because of organ shortage, donors who were initially excluded for various reasons have finally become acceptable since cold ischemia time can be prolonged in kidney transplantation without major changes in failure rate.

Extension of clinical indications for transplantation, along with the changes of donor and recipient populations, has raised unprecedented problems in evaluating a new protocol or a new immunosuppressive drug. Stratification of risk factors requires multiple trials among well-defined patient groups or, alternatively, very large multicenter trials with a retrospective demonstration of an equal distribution of all defined risk factors among the different groups. This is a major drawback since a large number of new chemical or biological agents derived from basic research require clinical evaluation while the number of organ transplantations performed each year remains stable. The shortage of organs and the satisfactory short term results raise ethical issues as to the acceptability of drastically new protocols of tolerance induction [1]. The risk of freezing the development of potential new drugs must be considered and the space left for innovation in transplantation appears to be extremely limited when compared to other fields of pharmacological research, e.g. antibiotics, cancer chemotherapy or cardiovascular drugs.

P. Cochat et al. (eds.), Immunosuppression under Trial, 169–178
©*1999 Kluwer Academic Publishers.*

Demonstrated or alleged risk factors and exclusion criteria in renal transplantation

Commonly identified risk factors in organ transplantation should be a cause of exclusion from trials of immunosuppressive agents because their incidence is likely to be uneven in small series, and because such risk factors use to have an individual approach according to each transplant center. The main risk factors in renal transplantation are listed in Table 1.

Differences in local policies primarily rely on the absence of consensus as to the precise impact of each risk factor. Hence donors with controlled infection or non-metastatic cancer are excluded by some groups but not by others. Some transplant centers reject organs from very young donors [2, 3] or from donors over 65 years of age whereas others rely on organ function assessment and sometimes biopsies [4–6] in order to decide whether organs can be transplanted [7–11]. Some centers allocate organs from elderly donors in age-matched recipients whereas others transplant two kidneys, instead of a single one. Organs from non-heart beating donors are used in a limited number of transplant centers.

Table 1.   Risk factors[a] in renal transplantation

Donor
  Age > 60
  Glomerulonephritis
  Cause of death (stroke)
  Cold ischemia > 36 or 48 h
  Non-heart-beating donor

Recipient
  Age < 5 or > 60
  Diabetes
  HLA antibodies > 80% of the panel
  Cardiovascular diseases
  Combined transplantation
  First graft lost from rejection
  HIV positive, active hepatitis
  Malignancy
  Non-compliance

Donor–recipient matching
  Sex (female to male)
  Size
  HLA DR mismatch
  Viral status (EBV$^+$ into EBV$^-$)

[a]Conditions associated with an increased risk of transplant failure or patient death, according to some reports. Many of these factors were also shown to allow satisfactory results when appropriately dealt with

No clear consensus has yet emerged as regards to the upper limit of warm and cold ischemia time. Although both experimental studies and clinical experience suggest that extending ischemia increases the risk of ischemic delayed graft function [12] and may subsequently compromise long-term graft function, no widely accepted guidelines are available, leading to marked differences in decision making among hospitals.

With respect to donor–recipient matching, there is a broad agreement on the need for improved HLA matching in hyperimmunized patients (in order to avoid a positive T cell cross-match), but opinions differ regarding better matching and increased immunosuppression for second heart or renal transplants [13]. Size matching in renal transplantation seems appropriate in order to avoid progressive renal insufficiency due to hyperfiltration in adult recipients of a small kidney. However, the relative influence of size matching versus other factors (e.g. HLA matching) on long-term results is not yet ascertained and no precise limit of size difference has been clearly demonstrated.

A less favourable outcome of female-to-male renal grafts has been reported [14] but the relative role of size mismatch [15] versus other factors such as drug toxicity is not precisely ascertained. The positive impact of HLA-DR matching is clearly documented in large series [12] but it may be compromised by cold ischemia time which accounts for an increased incidence of delayed graft function and subsequent late graft loss [12].

A long list of risk factors related to the recipients status has emerged from years of clinical practice. Interestingly some risks may be influenced by some specific advances in transplantation management. For instance primary cytomegalovirus infection was a cause of mortality in strongly immunosuppressed patients until the development of efficient antiviral therapy. Conversely lymphoproliferative disorders associated with Epstein-Barr virus remain a major complication of over-immunosuppression, especially in children who use to be seronegative and undergo primary infection in a state of iatrogenic T cell deficiency.

Cardiovascular diseases remain the main cause of death among transplant patients. However despite the fact that most cardiovascular risk factors are clearly identified and easily assessed prior to transplantation, major differences can be observed among centers regarding inclusion or exclusion of patients with such risks. The same holds true for patients with increased risk of non-compliance and those with various types of primary diseases leading to early (uropathies, vascular malformation) or delayed risk (recurrence of primary disease).

All risk factors shown to have a significant impact on patient or graft survival should be considered in the design of any immunosuppressive drug trial. An equal distribution of such factors in each arm of the trial must be retrospectively documented. Alternatively, demonstrated risk factors should be listed as exclusion factors. The former strategy is applicable to large-scale multicentre trials while the latter is suitable to smaller patient groups. However, such a rationale does not apply to current drug trials. Indeed exclusion factors from some recent trials (e.g. tacrolimus or CD25 monoclonal antibody) only partially overlaps with recognized risk factors (Table 2).

How to deal with risk factors in the design of drug trials?

Clinical trials are mandatory to demonstrate the efficacy of a new drug and considerable advances have been achieved in the approach of drug trial design. The number of patients enrolled may remain limited for new highly efficient drugs: after treating a few cases of tuberculosis meningitis with streptomycin the 'life and death' difference between treated and controls was so obvious that prolongation of a placebo-controlled trial would have been unethical. Major efficient drugs whose efficacy can be demonstrated in small series of patients may appear but their development is often hampered by the lack of a sizeable market and sufficient return on investment. Governmental agencies and European communities are looking for positive action to help pharmaceutical companies in order to compensate for the lack of profit in marketing those 'orphan drugs'. The vast majority of drug trials entail large series of patients because the expected benefit over existing therapies is often limited and the population of patients remains heterogeneous despite efforts of stratification.

When applied to immunosuppressive agents in organ transplantation the constraints of clinical evaluation may lead to two extreme strategies, using either large cohorts or small groups of patients. The former considers that most patients with recognized risk factors should be excluded from the trial (or alternatively, evenly distributed in the two groups, which considerably increases the size of the patient population). The latter strategy deals with clinical protocols designed for small groups of at-risk patients, such as diabetics or repeat grafts, or those in at-risk situations (elderly donors, long ischemia time). Such protocols are currently not encouraged for many reasons:

Table 2. Examples of exclusion criterias in clinical trials of immunosuppressive drugs

Living donor
Non-heart-beating donor/cold ischemia time > 48 h
Multiorgan recipients (e.g. kidney + pancreas)
HLA antibodies > 80% of the panel
Malignancy within the last 5 years
Pregnancy, lactation, non-acceptance of contraception
Mental dysfunction, risk of non compliance[a]
Age < 18 and > 60 or > 65
Second or third graft
Systemic disease treated with immunosuppressive drugs
Systemic infection, HIV positive, active hepatitis

[a]Several studies have shown that compliance is significantly improved when patients are enrolled in a trial

(1) manuscripts on significant results based on small series are rarely accepted in major journals;
(2) whatever its novelty, a drug whose activity is documented in a subgroup of at risk patients will remain an orphan drug;
(3) the increasing number of identified risk factors and their random combination in patient populations makes the definition of homogeneous subgroups quite impossible.

Although the current methodology for drug trials that requires large groups of organ recipients is mandatory for the clinical development of new immuno-suppressive drugs and their approval by regulation agencies, some obvious limitations and negative effects of this procedure should be briefly discussed, including methodological, ethical and public health issues.

Methodological and ethical issues of large scale drug trials in organ transplantation

The methodology of large scale clinical trials that are required to obtain evidence for potency and safety of a new immunosuppressive drug is well established [16–19]. The most common end-points are the incidence of acute rejection episodes [20] and transplant survival (or a certain level of transplant function) at one year. Simple end-points like serum creatinine at day 10 in association with at least one acute rejection episode may be a reliable indicator of cumulated risk factors and a good marker of prognosis [21]. In renal transplantation, collaborative efforts have led to a consensus on pathological criteria of allograft rejection (the Banff classification) [22]. It is well known by transplant clinicians, however, that many histologically mild rejection crises are spontaneously reversible. Furthermore, in several experimental models of tolerance induction long-term graft survival with normal function is achieved despite major mononuclear cell infiltration in the graft. Comparable obser-vations have been reported in various models of experimental type I (insulin-dependent) diabetes in which severe insulitis may develop in the absence of overt diabetes. Thus, a concept of 'rejection' versus 'no rejection', although valid for overt severe rejection episodes, is questionable and misleading when it includes moderate or mild crises. A similar debate arose as regards biopsy proven grades I and II rejection of heart transplants.

Another problem deals with the duration of the trial which is often limited to a one-year period. It is obvious that increasing initial immunosuppression will reduce the incidence of acute rejection episodes and possibly increase overall transplant survival at one year, but entails a greater risk of virus-associated neoplasia over the long term. The actual risk:benefit ratio of a new treatment can only be evaluated in the long term. This particularly applies to induction treatments and to new drugs which seem to be more efficient than the former ones (e.g. mycophenolate mofetil versus azathioprine).

A third methodological issue is the degree of inference that is acceptable from the conclusions of a trial. A drug whose activity has been tested at a given dose in association with certain other drugs in a standard population of low-risk patients will often be used at another dosage, with other drug combinations, even in high-risk patients who had been primarily excluded from the trial. The history of cyclosporin A shows that initial trials which were used to register the drug involved high dosages and unacceptable toxicity. A reduced incidence of cancer has been demonstrated by Dantal et al. by lowering the maintenance dosage of cyclosporin A with individual adjustment to blood levels [23, 24]. From these observations it is clear that governmental drug agencies should re-examine their policy with immunosuppressive agents and put even greater emphasis on pharmacovigilance, granting temporary approvals subject to ongoing evaluation including long-term effects.

Current drug trials may have an important yet unascertained effect on the overall management of organ transplantation. Most transplantation centers are eager to contribute to drug trials for obvious reasons (fame, better quality control, financial and technical assistance from pharmaceutical companies). However, because of organ shortage, there is a long waiting list for kidney grafts (median waiting time 2 years in France). The number of patients is therefore unsufficient to evaluate all the promising new molecules. The increasing population of at-risk patients raises major problems that outline the heterogeneity of policies among transplantation centers. In some centers or organ sharing institutions various categories of at-risk patients are regarded as a priority for organ allocation for ethical reasons, because their chances of survival without transplantation or their chances of finding a matched donor are rather poor (e.g. young children, diabetics, hyperimmunized patients). Such a policy will further restrict the number of low-risk patients available for drug trials. In other centers priority in allocation is given to low-risk patients in order to achieve an optimal use of transplants in a context of organ shortage. This may lead to major inequity in the waiting times for kidney transplants, ranging from 6 months to 10 years.

Finally the current emphasis on drug trials favours minor changes in management protocols and prevents the emergence of new strategies. Recent immunosuppressive agents may replace former drugs in a rather rigid scheme: CD25 antibody induction therapy instead of OKT3 or ATG, mycophenolate mofetil instead of azathioprine and tacrolimus instead of cyclosporin A. Such an empirical approach is supported neither by the analysis of molecular mechanisms of action nor by animal experiments. Protocols of tolerance induction that combine lymphocyte depletion or non-depleting antibodies with injection of anergizing donor cells are currently under development but their clinical application raises major difficulties. They should be attempted on small series of patients with fully informed consent and with alternative treatments available in case of failure (dialysis for renal transplant recipients). Such programs should be conducted in selected centers with an extensive experience of experimental models, after approval by an international board of experts.

Proposals for an integrated approach and their limitations

Clinical development of new treatments in organ transplantation is presently a field of conflict between diverging approaches that require global analysis and search for an agreement among all concerned physicians and institutions. The history of transplantation was built on a succession of challenges and bold attempts to demonstrate that lethal diseases could be treated by allografts. Transplant surgeons and physicians are reluctant to stick to an established routine and they are still eager to extend the field of transplantation. Research on xenografts is likely to bring important basic advances, to stimulate progress in biotechnology, but the dream of its rapid applicability to clinical transplantation should not hamper the clinical research on allografts. All efforts toward improvement of the management of high risk patients should be encouraged as well as clinical research in lung and small bowel transplantation.

Pharmaceutical companies are bound to discover and develop new drugs that can be marketed with a sufficient return on investment. At present the main costs in development are devoted to clinical trials. Evaluation of immuno-suppressive drugs is under a rigid methodology which does not take into consideration the rapid changes in patients' conditions, the emergence of new associated drugs, the long-term effects, and the possible drastic alterations that may be brought by tolerance induction. International companies should devote more funding to basic research. Furthermore it is their ethical responsibility to contribute to the long-term assessment and clinical monitoring of delayed effectiveness and side effects of immunosuppressive therapy (chronic rejection, tumors). In this respect, we must emphasize that the only end-points that matter in transplantation are survival, quality of life and optimal use of available resources, which do not rely on a single drug but on a whole therapeutic procedure, involving quality of the transplant, matching, surgical procedure, clinical monitoring and drug associations. Hence a policy focused on the rapid return on investment of a single drug may be misleading in the mid-term. Any progress in drug design will remain useless if the new drug is not properly integrated in the whole process from the onset of its development. However, no clear policy has yet emerged among major companies as regard trials of drug associations. Furthermore the multinational policy of drug companies imposed by registration and marketing constraints may not always fit patient needs and the allocation policies of national transplant associations.

From a public health and ethical viewpoint, all efforts should be devoted to ensure the most efficient use of the limited resources of organ donation. The major concerns are equity in the access to therapy and cost/benefit ratios. This implies that the results of transplantation should be evaluated by comparison with alternative treatments when available (dialysis versus transplantation in end stage renal failure, medical treatment versus transplantation in cardio-myopathies). In this respect, the problem of exclusion of high risk patients from renal transplantation should be discussed in the light of their survival rate on dialysis. In a situation of organ shortage it may not be ethical to compromise the chances of successful transplantation in low-risk patients by giving priority to high-risk patients, although such policy may be considered as ethical in the absence of organ shortage.

The responsibility of government agencies is to define a global policy integrating patients needs, pharmaceutical company constraints, ethics and public health objectives into a coherent approach. They should provide all epidemiological data pertinent to the global long-term assessment of therapies of any pathological condition that may require transplantation. They must ensure appropriate organ allocation and equity in access to the most efficient treatment. In addition, they should promote and coordinate therapeutical research and contribute to the funding of clinical protocols through contractual endeavours with insurance and pharmaceutical companies. To achieve this goal, it is mandatory that transplant agencies (e.g. Etablissement français des Greffes in France) promote a better coordination with drug administration agencies for a thorough evaluation of the adverse consequences of the present policies in drug registration in the field of transplantation. The present failure of such a coordination in France primarily relies on a restricted vision of the missions of each agency, a paradoxical yet not unique problem in a country where an historical tradition has endowed the state with a total control on trans-plantation but no mean to promote a coherent and synthetic policy.

Conclusion

In conclusion, the management of high risk patients in transplantation is a prototype of emerging problems in modern medicine. Conventional drug therapy relies on the definition of disease entities with common pathophysiological mechanisms and adapted drug treatments. Recent discoveries in immunology and genetics outline the major role of allelic polymorphism within the population in adaptative responses to environmental aggressions. The extreme diversity of individual genetic factors and their even higher combinatorial heterogeneity question the mere concept of disease entity, and provide a scientific basis for individually tailored therapies. Appropriate combinations of drugs whose activity has been demonstrated in conventional trials should be designed according to associated risk factors [13]. Future drug evaluation may rely on assessments within multiple subgroups of genetically defined at-risk patients rather than on an overall population study. It does not come as a surprise that rational efforts to promote scientifically evidence-based medicine remains a crude approach that is presently challenged by the discovery of allelic polymorphism of nearly all genes involved in adaptative responses.

Acknowledgements

P. Cochat is Professor of Pediatrics and Head of the pediatric renal unit (Hôpital Edouard Herriot, Lyon). C. Pouteil-Noble, Professor of Nephrology and Head of the renal transplantation unit (Centre Hospitalier Lyon-Sud, Hospices Civils de Lyon). J.P. Revillard is presently Head of the immunopharmacology unit, INSERM U.503 Lyon. This study was supported by INSERM, Claude Bernard University, Région Rhône-Alpes and Fondation pour la Recherche Médicale.

References

1. Pearson TC, Madsen JC, Larsen CP, Morris PJ, Wood KJ. Induction of transplantation tolerance in adults using donor antigen and anti-CD4 monoclonal antibody. Transplantation. 1992; 54: 475–483.
2. Genyk Y, Knight R, Burrows L. Should pediatric donors younger than 2 years of age be used in kidney transplantation? Transplant. Proc. 1997; 29: 3276–3277.
3. Banowsky LH, Lackner J, Kothmann R, Wright F. Results of single kidneys from donors aged 9 to 60 months: results in 144 adult recipients. Transplant. Proc. 1997; 29: 3271–3273.
4. Abdi R, Slakey D, Kittur D, Burkick J, Racusen L. Baseline glomerular size as a predictor of function in human renal transplantation. Transplantation. 1998; 66: 329–333.
5. Cosyns JP, Malaise J, Hanique G, Mourad M, Baldi A, Goebbels RM, Squifflet JP. Lesions in donor kidneys: nature, incidence, and influence on graft function. Transplant. Int. 1998; 11: 22–27.
6. Gaber LW, Moore LW, Alloway RR, Amiri MH, Vera SR, Gaber AO. Glomerulosclerosis as a determinant of posttransplant function of older donor renal allografts. Transplantation. 1995; 60: 334–339.
7. Higgins RM, Sheriff R, Bittar AA, Richardson AJ, Ratcliffe PJ, Gray DWR, Morris PJ. The quality of function of renal allografts is associated with donor age. Transplant. Int. 1995; 8: 221–225.
8. Terasaki PI, Gjertson DW, Cecka JM, Takemoto S, Cho YW. Significance of the donor age effect on kidney transplants. Clin. Transplant. 1997; 11: 366–372.
9. Abouna GM. Marginal donors: a viable solution for organ shortage. Transplant. Proc. 1997; 29: 2759–2764.
10. Anil Kumar MS, Panigrahi D, Dezii CM et al. Long-term function and survival of elderly donor kidneys transplanted into young adults. Transplantation. 1998; 65: 282–285.
11. Sola R, Guirado LL, Lopez Navidad A et al. Renal transplantation with limit donors. Transplantation. 1998; 66: 1159–1163.
12. Connolly JK, Dyer PA, Martin S, Parrott NR, Pearson RC, Johnson RWG. Importance of minimizing HLA-DR mismatch and cold preservation time in cadaveric renal transplantation. Transplantation. 1996; 61: 709–714.
13. Robertson AJ, Morris PJ. Do re-grafts require more aggressive immunosuppression? Transplant. Clin. Immunol. 1997; 29: 109–119.
14. Neugarten J, Srinivas T, Tellis V, Silbiger S, Greenstein S. The effect of donor gender on renal allograft survival. J. Am. Soc. Nephrol. 1996; 7: 318–324.
15. Miles AMV, Sumrani N, John S et al. The effect of kidney size on cadaveric renal allograft outcome. Transplantation. 1996; 61: 894–897.
16. Mirsch JD, Miller J, Deierhoi MH, Vincenti F, Filo RS for the FK506 kidney transplant study group. A comparison of tacrolimus (FK506) and cyclosporine for immunosuppression after cadaveric renal transplantation. Transplantation. 1997; 63: 977–83.
17. Mayer AD, Dmitrewski J, Squifflet JP et al. Multicenter randomized trial comparing

tacrolimus (FK506) and cyclosporine in the prevention of renal allograft rejection. A report of the European tacrolimus multicenter renal study group. Transplantation. 1997; 64: 436–443.

18. Sollinger HN. Mycophenolate mofetil for the prevention of acute rejection in primary cadaveric renal allograft recipients. Transplantation. 1995; 60: 225–232.

19. Halloran P, Mathew T, Tomlanovich S, Groth C, Hooftman L, Barker C for the international mycophenolate mofetil renal transplant study group. Mycophenolate mofetil in allograft recipients. Transplantation. 1997; 63: 39–47.

20. Gulanickar AC, McDonald AC. Sungertekin U, Belitsky P. The incidence and impact of early rejection episodes on graft outcome in recipients of first cadaver kidney transplants. Transplantation. 1992; 53: 323.

21. Pfaff WW, Howard RJ, Patton PR, Adams VR, Rosen CB, Reed AI. Delayed graft function after renal transplantation. Transplantation. 1998; 65: 219–223.

21. Cosio FG, Pelletier RP, Falkenhain ME et al. Impact of acute rejection and early allograft function on renal allograft survival. Transplantation. 1997; 63: 1611–1615.

22. Solez K. Axelsen RA, Benekiktsson H et al. International standardization of criteria for the histologic diagnosis of renal allograft rejection: the Banff working classification of kidney transplant pathology. Kidney Int. 1993; 44: 411–422.

23. Newstead CG. Assessment of risk of cancer renal transplantation. Lancet. 1998; 351: 610–611.

24. Dantal J, Hourmant M, Cantarovitch D, Giral M, Blancho G, Dreno B, Soulillou JP. Effect of long-term immunosuppression in kidney-graft recipients on cancer incidence: randomised comparison of two cyclosporin regimens. Lancet. 1998; 351: 623–628.

Name Index